Practicing in the Age of AI

Essays on Medicine, Meaning, and Machines

Arthur Lazarus, MD, MBA, CPE, DFAAPL

AAPL

978-1-960762-65-8 print
978-1-960762-66-5 eBook

Published by **American Association for Physician Leadership, Inc.**
PO Box 96503 | BMB 97493 | Washington, DC 20090-6503

Website: www.physicianleaders.org

AAPL books are available at special quantity discounts to use as premiums and sales promotions, or for use in corporate training programs. For more information, please write to Special Sales at journal@physicianleaders.org

This publication is designed to provide general information and is sold with the understanding that neither the author nor the publisher is engaged in rendering legal, accounting, ethical, or clinical advice. If legal or other expert advice is required, the services of a competent professional person should be sought.

13 8 7 6 5 4 3 2 1

Copyedited, typeset, indexed, and printed in the United States of America

PUBLISHER
Nancy Collins

PRODUCTION MANAGER
Jennifer Weiss

DESIGN & LAYOUT
Carter Publishing Studio

COPYEDITOR
Patricia George

NOTE TO READERS

THE ESSAYS IN THIS BOOK are grounded in observation, reflection, research, and my experience as a physician writing about medicine in the age of artificial intelligence. Thirty-three are nonfiction essays offered in that spirit; three — essays 9, 20, and 31 — use fictionalized or composite elements to explore real tensions in contemporary practice. In those three essays, any resemblance to actual persons, living or dead, or to real events is coincidental.

Website links are included in some references. I've done my best to ensure they were accurate at the time of writing, but online addresses change, move, or disappear over time. If a link no longer works, a quick search by title will usually lead you to an updated source.

I used ChatGPT and Doximity Ask, OpenAI GPT-based model (a HIPAA-compliant AI assistant designed for U.S. healthcare professionals) as editorial aids to assist with language refinement, clarity, and research navigation. All ideas, structure, narrative voice, and final content are my own, and I retain full responsibility for the accuracy, integrity, and originality of the material presented.

This book contains discussions of suicide and suicidal behavior. If you or someone you know is struggling with suicidal thoughts or self-harming behaviors, call or text 988 to get help from the 988 Suicide & Crisis Lifeline.

Nothing in this book is intended as medical advice or a substitute for professional medical care. The reflections, opinions, and observations expressed here are offered to provoke thought and discussion, not to provide diagnosis or treatment.

ALSO BY ARTHUR LAZARUS

NONFICTION

Neuroleptic Malignant Syndrome and Related Conditions (co-author)

Controversies in Managed Mental Health Care

Career Pathways in Psychiatry: Transition in Changing Times

MD/MBA: Physicians on the New Frontier of Medical Management

Every Story Counts: Exploring Contemporary Practice Through Narrative Medicine

Medicine on Fire: A Narrative Travelogue

Narrative Medicine: The Fifth Vital Sign

Narrative Medicine: Harnessing the Power of Storytelling through Essays

Story Treasures: Medical Essays and Insights in the Narrative Tradition

21st Century Schizoid Health Care: Essays and Reflections to Keep You Sane on Your Medical Travels

Narrative Rx: A Quick Guide to Narrative Medicine for Students, Residents, and Attendings

Narrative Medicine: New and Selected Essays

Narrative Frontiers: Essays at the Edge of Medicine and the Multiverse

Critical Condition: American Medicine at the Quarter-Century Mark

How to Jumpstart Your Medical Career and Thrive in Practice: Practical Advice and Insight from a Battle-Tested Physician

Still Life with Stethoscope and Typewriter: Essays and Echoes of Narrative Medicine

Narrative Medicine in the Age of Uncertainty: Where Systems Strain and Stories Steady

Nobody Told Me There'd Be Days Like These: Hard Truths from Physicians — and What They Mean for Medical Practice

FICTION

Born to Heal: Medical Narratives Set to the Soundtrack of Classic Rock

Real Medicine, Unreal Stories: Lessons and Insights from Clinical Practice (Volumes 1-6)

Rounds Never End: Three Tales of Medicine, Deception, and Discovery (Volumes 1&2)

Standard of Care: Medical Judgment on Trial

Against the Tide: A Doctor's Battle for an Undocumented Patient

Jailbreak: When Artificial Intelligence Breaks Medicine

Transplant: A Novel

The Body Brokers: Inside Medicine's Referral and Discharge Machinery

The New Eugenics in Medicine: Two Novellas About Power, Science, and the Future of Human Worth

The Semmelweis Effect: When Medicine Knows Harm Exists — and Proceeds Anyway

Sick and Systemic: Absurd Scenes from a Medical System That Works — Just Not for You (Volumes 1-4)

TABLE OF CONTENTS

About the Author

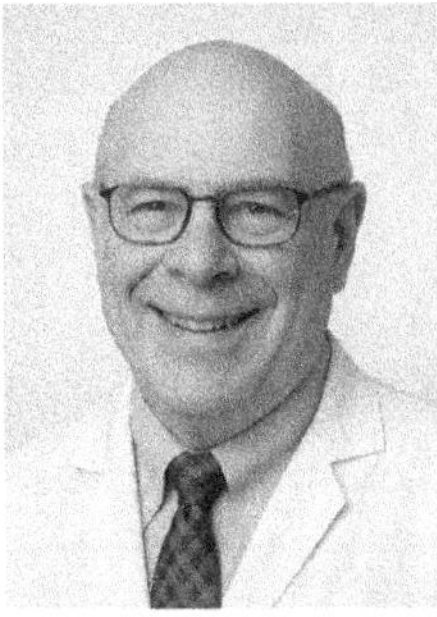

Arthur Lazarus, MD, MBA, is a healthcare consultant, certified physician executive, and nationally recognized author, speaker, and champion of physician leadership and wellness. He has broad experience in clinical practice and the health insurance industry, having led programs at Cigna and Humana. At Humana, Lazarus was vice president and corporate medical director of behavioral health operations in Louisville, Kentucky, and subsequently a population health medical director in the state of Florida.

Lazarus has also held leadership positions in several pharmaceutical companies, including Pfizer and AstraZeneca, supervising clinical trials and reviewing promotional material for medical accuracy and FDA compliance.

With over 500 articles and essays across scientific journals, professional publications, and online platforms, Lazarus has built a wide-ranging literary presence. He is the author of numerous books on narrative medicine and is the creator of the acclaimed fictional series *Rounds Never End* and *Real Medicine, Unreal Stories*. His writing focuses on the forces reshaping modern medicine — from burnout and bias to technology, ethics, and the enduring power of narrative.

Born in Philadelphia, Pennsylvania, Lazarus attended Boston University, where he graduated with a bachelor's degree in psychology with distinction. He received his medical degree with honors from the Lewis Katz School of Medicine at Temple University, followed by a psychiatric residency at Temple University Hospital, where he was chief resident.

After residency, Lazarus joined the faculty of Temple's Lewis Katz School of Medicine, where he currently serves as adjunct professor of psychiatry. He also holds non-faculty appointments as executive-in-residence at Temple University Fox School of Business and Management, where he received his MBA degree, and senior fellow, Jefferson College of Population Health, Philadelphia, Pennsylvania.

Well known for his leadership and medical management skills, Lazarus is a sought-after presenter, mentor, teacher, and writer. He has shared his expertise and perspective at numerous local, national, and international meetings and seminars.

Lazarus is a past president of the American Association for Psychiatric Administration and Leadership, a distinguished fellow of the American Association for Physician Leadership (AAPL), and a current member of the AAPL editorial review board. In 2010, the American Psychiatric Association honored Lazarus with the Administrative Psychiatry Award for his effectiveness as an administrator of major mental health programs and for expanding the body of knowledge of management science in mental health services delivery systems.

Lazarus is among a select group of physicians in the United States who have been inducted into both the Alpha Omega Alpha medical honor society and the Beta Gamma Sigma honor society of collegiate schools of business.

Beyond medicine, Lazarus enjoys walking, biking, playing piano, and listening to music. He and his wife Cheryl have four grown children and seven grandchildren. They live in Asheville, North Carolina.

Introduction

Medicine has always been shaped by its tools. The stethoscope changed how physicians listened. The microscope changed how we saw disease. Imaging technologies allowed us to peer inside the living body without a scalpel. Each innovation expanded medicine's reach while forcing clinicians to reconsider what it meant to practice thoughtfully and responsibly. Artificial intelligence is the newest and perhaps most consequential addition to that lineage.

Across hospitals, laboratories, and clinics, AI is no longer a future possibility but a present reality. Machine learning algorithms analyze medical images, detect patterns in vast data sets, and predict clinical outcomes with increasing accuracy. Natural language processing systems assist with documentation and patient communication. Large language models summarize research, draft notes, and synthesize complex clinical information. What once seemed futuristic has become embedded in the everyday infrastructure of care.

This transformation is not a rupture but an acceleration. Medicine has always been data-rich. A single patient generates layers of information, including history, laboratory results, imaging studies, pathology, genomics, and environmental context. All of this must be interpreted together. As healthcare digitized and complexity increased, the volume of data outpaced any individual clinician's capacity to synthesize it alone. Artificial intelligence emerged, in part, as a response to that reality.

Modern AI systems excel at large-scale pattern recognition. They identify relationships that may escape human detection and extend medicine's analytical reach across disciplines. Their applications now span diagnosis, clinical decision support, workflow, and research. In parallel, the vision of personalized medicine, care tailored to each patient's biological and environmental profile, has moved closer to feasibility. The promise is compelling: medicine that is more precise, anticipatory, and efficient.

But enthusiasm must be tempered by realism.

Algorithms learn from data that often reflect existing inequities. Underrepresentation can propagate diagnostic error and widen disparities. Many systems function as "black boxes," generating outputs without transparent reasoning. Questions of privacy, data ownership, cybersecurity, and regulatory oversight remain unsettled. When AI contributes to error, accountability is often unclear. These are not merely technical problems. They are ethical and philosophical ones.

Artificial intelligence challenges long-standing assumptions about expertise, judgment, and responsibility. When algorithms offer probabilistic guidance, how should clinicians weigh that advice? When machines increasingly participate in the cognitive work of medicine, what remains uniquely human about the practice of healing?

Even when AI is not explicitly invoked, it shapes the environment in which care is delivered. Algorithms triage imaging studies, predictive models populate electronic records, and automated systems influence documentation and work processes. AI is no longer a discrete tool. It is an ambient condition of contemporary medicine.

Some clinicians experience this shift as liberation from administrative burden. Others see it as a threat to professional autonomy. The future will likely reflect neither extreme. Artificial intelligence is unlikely to replace physicians, but it will reshape what physicians do. Increasingly, the clinician's role may evolve from primary generator of medical knowledge to editor, interpreter, and steward of machine-assisted insight.

Practicing in the Age of AI explores this evolving relationship through a collection of essays examining how artificial intelligence is reshaping medicine technologically, culturally, and philosophically. Some essays focus on specific applications, including documentation, diagnostics, decision support, and research. Others examine broader consequences, such as automation bias, fabricated outputs, algorithmic inequity, and the subtle ways AI reshapes language, thought, and professional identity.

Readers may notice that certain ideas recur across multiple essays, including scalability, workflow, ecosystem, governance, trust, and judgment. This repetition is intentional. Artificial intelligence is complex and rapidly evolving. Understanding its implications requires revisiting core concepts from different angles. By encountering them across clinical examples, ethical dilemmas, and narrative reflections, the reader gains not only familiarity with AI's capabilities but a deeper understanding of the themes that define its impact on medicine.

Several of those themes appear throughout the book:

- As AI changes medicine, it will change how we write and how we think.
- When machines speak with authority, trust becomes reflexive, but caution must remain.
- AI will not replace physicians; it will augment them when implemented thoughtfully.
- Ultimately, the future of AI in medicine will be determined not by capability alone, but by the values that guide it.

At its core, this book explores a central tension: medicine as a computational enterprise versus medicine as a human practice. Artificial intelligence thrives on statistical relationships. Medicine unfolds in stories. Each patient encounter is shaped by experience, meaning, and context. These elements resist full quantification.

AI may help us see more clearly, analyze more deeply, and act more efficiently. The essential tasks of medicine, however, remain human. These include interpreting evidence, navigating uncertainty, communicating with empathy, and assuming responsibility. If the age of AI demands anything of medicine, it is clarity about what cannot be delegated.

Accordingly, these essays focus less on the technology itself and more on those affected by it. This includes clinicians, trainees, researchers, policy leaders, technologists, and patients. In short, anyone interested in how machines are entering the spaces where care is delivered.

The book unfolds along a natural progression. It begins with language and thought, examining how AI shapes writing, communication, and clinical cognition. It then moves into practice, where tools reshape workflow, documentation, education, and the physician's role. From there, it turns to trust, authority, and the human stakes of AI in medicine, where error, empathy, and professional identity come into sharper focus. Finally, it steps back to consider the broader system, including policy, structure, and the future direction of a profession increasingly shaped by intelligent machines.

I did not set out to write a blueprint for fixing healthcare but rather a framework for understanding how it is changing. The question is no longer whether AI will shape medicine (it already does). The deeper question is how medicine will shape AI and, in doing so, preserve its human core within a transformed landscape.

Section I.

The Writing Mind Meets the Machine

Essay 1.

What Does the "A" in AI Stand For — Artificial or Augmented? The Case of Medical Writing

Artificial intelligence (AI) is reshaping healthcare, and medical writing sits squarely in its path of transformation. What began as spell-checkers and keyword searches now includes systems that summarize dense literature in minutes, suggest study rationales, draft plain-language summaries, check statistical coherence, and flag inconsistent reporting.

For clinicians, researchers, and professional writers who must synthesize complex evidence under time pressure, AI offers leverage: It accelerates routine work, brings structure to messy information, and can nudge prose toward clarity and reader-friendliness.

Yet AI does not replace fundamental scholarly judgment. Medical writing is not merely the arrangement of words; it is the responsible interpretation of data, alignment with standards of evidence, and transparent communication tailored to clinicians, regulators, patients, and the public.

Used well, AI can improve efficiency, accuracy, and reach. Used naively, it can introduce subtle errors, conceal bias in a fluent voice, or compromise confidentiality. The question, therefore, is not simply whether AI will participate in medical writing. It already does. The deeper question is what the "A" in AI ultimately represents in practice.

Is it **Artificial** intelligence replacing human work?

Or **Augmented** intelligence supporting it?

The answer, at least for now, lies in the tension between the two.

The Expanding Toolkit of Medical Writing

Artificial intelligence refers broadly to computer systems designed to perform tasks that typically require human intelligence: recognizing patterns, making predictions, and using language in context. Within this broad field, three concepts are particularly relevant to medical writers.

1. **Machine learning** encompasses algorithms that learn from data to make predictions or classifications. In writing, this capacity powers document clustering, relevance ranking, and error detection.
2. **Natural language processing (NLP)** is a subset of AI that enables computers to interpret, generate, and manipulate human language. It underpins tasks such as concept extraction, summarization, and translation.
3. **Large language models (LLMs)** — systems such as Generative Pre-trained Transformer (GPT)-based models — extend NLP further by generating fluent, contextually relevant text after being trained on vast amounts of written material. For medical writers, these models can assist in drafting sections of manuscripts, converting technical details into plain language, or harmonizing style across contributions from multiple authors.

A functional grasp of these ideas helps writers select tools wisely and understand where AI excels and where human expertise remains indispensable.

The integration of technology into medical writing has followed a steady trajectory over several decades. In the mid-20th century, tools such as *Index Medicus* and later PubMed revolutionized information retrieval, shifting literature searches from manual index cards to electronic databases. Early computer-assisted writing support was limited to spell-checking and grammar correction, which, though modest, marked the beginning of automated quality control in scholarly communication. By the early 2000s, reference managers such as EndNote and RefWorks began to ease the burden of citation formatting and bibliographic organization.

The most recent paradigm shift has come with NLP and large language models. Unlike earlier tools that primarily assisted with mechanics, these systems can now generate coherent drafts, translate text across languages, and even enforce elements of reporting standards. In this sense, the current wave of AI represents not just an incremental advance but a qualitative transformation in the scope of automation available to medical writers.

Understanding this historical progression contextualizes both the opportunities and challenges posed by today's AI systems.

When "Artificial" Sounds Tempting

For anyone who has spent long nights assembling manuscripts, regulatory submissions, or systematic reviews, the promise of artificial intelligence can feel almost miraculous. A literature search that once required hours of filtering can now be summarized in minutes. Draft outlines appear instantly. Tables populate themselves. Language that once required multiple revisions arrives already polished.

In the abstract, the appeal is obvious. If AI can write competently, why not allow it to write entirely?

The reason is that medicine has often painfully learned that efficiency alone is not the highest value in scientific communication. Medical writing exists not merely to produce text, but to represent truth responsibly. Data must be interpreted within context. Statistical claims must align with methods. Conclusions must match evidence. Language must remain faithful to uncertainty, nuance, and limitation.

An algorithm may produce sentences. Only a trained writer can ensure those sentences are ethically and scientifically justified.

When AI drafts prose without careful oversight, the risk is not only error but illusory authority. The writing sounds confident. The logic appears smooth. But subtle distortions can slip through unnoticed: a misplaced inference, a fabricated citation, a statistical interpretation that appears plausible but is fundamentally incorrect. The danger lies precisely in AI's strength: its fluency.

A machine that writes awkwardly invites scrutiny. A machine that writes beautifully may escape it.

The Case for Augmentation

Seen from this perspective, the more productive interpretation of AI in medical writing is not artificial replacement, but intellectual augmentation. AI can relieve writers of the mechanical burdens that historically consumed disproportionate time: formatting references, structuring sections, checking consistency across long documents, or converting dense material into accessible summaries.

These are tasks that benefit from computational speed but still require human verification. When used thoughtfully, AI becomes a cognitive exoskeleton, supporting the writer's capacity rather than supplanting it.

A clinician writing a review article might use AI to:

- Summarize a set of relevant papers.
- Suggest structural outlines.
- Translate technical material into plain-language summaries.
- Flag inconsistencies across draft sections.

But the clinician must still decide:

- Which studies matter.
- What the evidence truly shows.
- How limitations should be framed.
- Whether the final narrative reflects the literature honestly.

In other words, AI can assist with expression, but human expertise remains responsible for interpretation.

The Ethical Boundary

Medical writing carries obligations that extend beyond technical accuracy. Scientific communication affects regulatory decisions, clinical practice guidelines, patient expectations, and public trust. Even subtle distortions can influence treatment choices, policy debates, or perceptions of safety. For that reason, the ethical framework surrounding AI-assisted writing matters deeply.

Several principles have begun to emerge across journals and regulatory bodies:

Transparency. Authors should disclose meaningful AI assistance in drafting or editing text.

Accountability. The named authors remain responsible for all content, regardless of AI involvement.

Verification. AI-generated claims, citations, and interpretations must be independently validated.

Confidentiality. Sensitive patient information or unpublished data should not be exposed to external AI systems without appropriate safeguards.

These guardrails do not prohibit AI use. They simply acknowledge that scientific authorship carries responsibility that cannot be delegated to software.

The Subtle Transformation of Writing

Even when AI is used responsibly, it may still influence how medical writing evolves. Writers increasingly interact with AI as a collaborative drafting partner (see Essay 2). Writing prompts, as discussed in Essay 14, function as instructions that translate human intent into structured AI output. Iterative revisions occur through dialogue with a system that proposes alternative phrasings or reorganizes content.

This changes the rhythm of writing. The process becomes less solitary and more iterative, less about constructing every sentence from scratch and more about shaping and refining generated material.

In many ways, this resembles earlier technological shifts. Word processors once replaced typewriters. Reference managers replaced index cards. Electronic databases replaced library stacks. Each innovation altered the mechanics of writing without fundamentally changing its intellectual core.

AI may represent a more powerful version of the same trajectory. But the underlying work, the judgment that determines what should be written, remains human.

The Enduring Role of the Writer

Ultimately, the defining feature of medical writing is not the production of language but the curation of meaning.

A good medical writer does several things that no algorithm fully replicates:

- Evaluates the credibility of evidence.
- Understands the clinical implications of findings.
- Anticipates how readers will interpret claims.
- Communicates uncertainty honestly.

These tasks depend on experience, ethical awareness, and contextual knowledge. They require more than linguistic fluency. They require professional responsibility.

In this sense, the future of AI in medical writing may resemble the future of calculators in mathematics. Calculators did not eliminate mathematicians. They eliminated tedious arithmetic so that mathematicians could focus on deeper reasoning.

AI may perform a similar function for writing. It can draft. It can summarize. It can reorganize. But it cannot bear responsibility for what is ultimately put on paper.

Artificial or Augmented?

So, what does the "A" in AI truly stand for in medical writing?

If we imagine AI as a replacement for scholarly judgment, then the answer would be **Artificial** — a synthetic intelligence-producing text that only resembles understanding.

But if we see AI as a tool that expands human capability while leaving interpretation, ethics, and responsibility firmly in human hands, the answer becomes **Augmented**.

Artificial intelligence can generate sentences. Augmented intelligence helps writers think more clearly. Medical writing requires the latter. Because writing in medicine is not merely the production of text. It is the interpretation of evidence, the weighing of uncertainty, and the acceptance of responsibility for what enters the scientific record. That responsibility remains the province of human intelligence.

Essay 2.

Tools, Applications, and Ethical Considerations in AI-Assisted Medical and Scientific Writing

AI can play a role at nearly every stage of the medical writing process. One area of particular value is literature searching and review. AI-enabled platforms can scan enormous collections of abstracts and full-text articles, group them by themes, and generate preliminary summaries.

This capacity makes it easier to scope the literature quickly, identify gaps, and prepare evidence maps that clarify where data are strong or sparse. However, these systems can still miss crucial papers or overemphasize highly cited studies, underscoring the need for traditional searching and human oversight.

Drafting and editing manuscripts has also been transformed. Large language models can generate outlines, suggest ways to sharpen topic sentences, and harmonize tone in collaborative projects. Some tools specialize in polishing specific sections, such as methods or discussion, or in producing lay summaries and abstracts. While these capabilities save time, they also carry the risk of introducing fabricated references or unsupported claims. Writers, therefore, must carefully verify all AI-generated content.

Another domain is data analysis and visualization. AI systems can detect patterns, highlight outliers, and translate statistical outputs into prose that is accessible to readers. They can also help generate clear, well-labeled figures and tables. Yet even here, statistical expertise is indispensable to confirm the validity of the analyses.

Reference management has benefited from AI as well. Modern reference managers can automatically suggest missing citations, resolve duplicates, and ensure proper formatting according to journal style guides. They can even cross-check that each citation appears correctly in text and in the reference list. Still, metadata should always be verified against authoritative databases.

Language translation and accessibility represent additional gains. Neural translation systems produce increasingly accurate first drafts of translated documents, enabling greater global collaboration. Similarly, AI can convert technical text into plain-language summaries suitable for patients and policymakers. Such tools, however, must be used with caution, as nuance can be lost or misinterpreted.

Finally, plagiarism detection has become more sophisticated through AI. Similarity-checking software not only identifies verbatim overlap but also detects paraphrase plagiarism and formulaic writing. Authors can use these insights to revise and ensure their work maintains originality and integrity.

Education and Career Implications

The impact of AI on medical writing varies with the stage of a clinician's career. Medical students may first encounter AI when drafting case reports or reflective essays. Tools can support language refinement and adherence to journal formatting, though students must learn to evaluate the accuracy of suggested content. Residents and fellows, often writing under time pressure, can leverage AI to scope literature and draft abstracts while retaining responsibility for data integrity and interpretation.

For early-career faculty, AI offers advantages in grant writing and systematic reviews. Automated screening platforms can accelerate evidence synthesis, while LLMs can generate lay summaries for community engagement sections of grants. At the senior faculty and leadership levels, AI tools may be particularly helpful in preparing consensus statements, guidelines, and editorials — documents that require balancing technical precision with readability for diverse audiences.

Framing AI across these career stages underscores its role as an evolving partner: a language scaffold for novices, a productivity enhancer for mid-career clinicians, and a communication aid for senior professionals. In every case, the clinician's role shifts from producing raw text to curating, verifying, and ethically shaping AI outputs.

Clinicians can also shape AI from an overly agreeable *hype man* into a constructive *sparring partner* by using structured prompts that force multiple perspectives. A simple triad requesting (1) a neutral, unbiased appraisal; (2) a devil's-advocate critique that surfaces logical gaps, overclaims, or missing evidence; and (3) an encouraging, solutions-oriented view balancing support with rigor. Applied at different career stages, this method helps students stress-test case reports, residents pressure-check abstracts, junior faculty harden grant aims, and senior authors interrogate guideline language.

AI can also be used to pressure-test career decisions and choices. Consider this example, a query to ChatGPT:

You: I'm thinking of quitting my medical career tomorrow to become a full-time novelist.

ChatGPT: That sounds amazing! If writing excites you, it could be such a fulfilling path. Your medical background will give your stories a unique edge, and you deserve to chase what inspires you. Go for it!

Here's the "triad" applied to ChatGPT's overly enthusiastic response:

1. Neutral, Unbiased View

The response is supportive and encouraging, but it lacks balance. It highlights the potential fulfillment of a writing career but does not acknowledge the risks of abruptly leaving medicine or the practical considerations involved. The language is conversational and motivational, rather than analytical or cautious.

2. Devil's Advocate View

Quitting medicine "tomorrow" to pursue novel writing could be financially and emotionally destabilizing. A medical career is difficult to rebuild if abandoned abruptly. Many writers struggle for years before achieving a sustainable income. By cheerleading without caveats, the AI risks trivializing the gravity of leaving a highly trained profession. A better response would raise questions: Can you test the waters part-time? Do you have financial security? Will you miss the identity and purpose medicine provides?

3. Encouraging, Positive View

The response captures a valid truth: Pursuing passion can be deeply rewarding. A medical background gives a unique vantage point for compelling storytelling, and few novelists have lived the realities of patient care, ethics, and health systems. If writing truly excites you, nurturing that path (even gradually) could enrich your life and contribute something valuable to readers. Framing your medical experience as a strength may give you a distinctive literary voice.

The original AI reply was too one-dimensional. Applying the triad framework turns it into a richer, more useful reflection: acknowledge the appeal, raise the risks, and suggest realistic next steps. The practical takeaway is to read the devil's-advocate output with special care and learn how to prompt AI for the best results.

AI Tools and Platforms for Medical Writers

Several categories of AI tools are available to support medical writers. Writing assistants, such as Grammarly and GPT-based systems, offer grammar, style, and clarity enhancements. Systematic review platforms, including Covidence and Rayyan, employ machine learning to expedite abstract screening and data extraction. Reference managers, such as EndNote, Zotero, and Mendeley, increasingly integrate AI features for citation management and journal recommendations.

Plagiarism detection tools, including Turnitin and iThenticate, remain widely used for ensuring originality. Finally, publisher-side submission systems are beginning to deploy AI for checking formatting, reporting guideline compliance, and verifying ethics prior to peer review.

When selecting among these options, medical writers should prioritize tools that preserve transparency, maintain secure handling of confidential material, and integrate smoothly with existing workflows. Further discussion of AI tools is presented in Essay 12.

Integrating AI into the Medical Writing Workflow

AI can be introduced at virtually any stage of the writing process. During the earliest phases, writers may use it to brainstorm research questions, identify gaps in the literature, or generate possible titles and outlines. During drafting, AI can assist by producing first-pass text, whether for an introduction, background, or abstract, based on user-supplied material.

In the revision phase, writers often employ AI to smooth language, harmonize terminology, and check grammar or style. Later, at the submission stage, AI can confirm compliance with journal formatting rules and highlight areas where reporting standards are not fully met.

An example illustrates the potential of this integrated approach. Imagine a clinician preparing a grant proposal. They begin by using an AI-powered literature review platform to identify and categorize recent studies. Next, they rely on a large language model to draft the background section, drawing on those identified papers. A reference manager formats and organizes citations, while plagiarism-detection software verifies originality. At each step, the clinician reviews and refines, ensuring accuracy and nuance. The end product is a polished, ethically sound proposal completed more efficiently than by traditional means.

In writing this essay, I used AI sparingly to support the refinement process. After I created an outline and wrote the content for each section, I employed ChatGPT to suggest improvements in clarity, style, and flow. AI also assisted in the generation of source material; however, all content or interpretations suggested by ChatGPT was reviewed, verified, and edited by me to ensure accuracy. The checklist at the end of this essay guided my use of AI in preparing it.

Benefits and Limitations of AI in Medical Writing

AI offers significant advantages in medical writing. These systems improve efficiency by automating repetitive tasks such as formatting references or screening literature, allowing writers to focus on analysis and interpretation. They also enhance accuracy by reducing typographical errors, inconsistencies, and formatting mistakes. Moreover, AI systems scale easily, handling large volumes of information and facilitating projects like systematic reviews or living guidelines that demand ongoing updating.

Despite these strengths, AI has clear limitations. One challenge is the tendency of large language models to generate so-called "hallucinations," or plausible-sounding but false information. Another is the risk of perpetuating bias, since models often reflect the distributions and inequities present in their training data.

Furthermore, AI frequently lacks the subtle domain-specific judgment that medical writing requires, particularly when interpreting ambiguous data or balancing competing perspectives. For these reasons, human review and accountability remain essential.

Ethical, Legal, and Professional Considerations

The integration of AI into medical writing raises important ethical questions. Authorship is one such area. AI is a tool, not a responsible agent, and therefore cannot qualify as an author under guidelines such as those of the International Committee of Medical Journal Editors. Human writers must remain accountable for accuracy and integrity, while disclosures about AI use are increasingly required.

Data privacy and confidentiality represent another critical concern. Writers must ensure that no protected health information (PHI) or proprietary data are uploaded to AI systems, particularly those that process content in the cloud. Secure platforms and de-identification are essential safeguards.

As mentioned, plagiarism and scientific integrity are paramount and demand vigilance. While AI can help generate original text, writers must confirm that all claims are supported by evidence and that paraphrasing reflects genuine understanding rather than superficial rewording.

Compliance with institutional, journal, and funding policies is imperative. Many organizations now issue guidance on acceptable uses of AI in manuscript preparation. Transparency — detailing which tools were used and how — remains the safest and most ethical approach. Notably, the U.S. Copyright Office does not recognize AI as an author.

Finally, authors must never take credit for a work written by AI. It's lazy and disingenuous at best, and dishonest and unethical at worst. Letting AI "do the job" negates the writer's authentic voice and eliminates critical thinking skills. In medicine, especially in a learning environment involving trainees, overuse of AI may produce expert opinions while failing to produce experts. Students may not even retain a memory of the final product they claim as their own because they were never fully engaged in its creation.

A 2025 study by researchers at the MIT Media Lab found that heavy reliance on AI tools like ChatGPT for tasks such as essay writing is associated with reduced brain activity.[1] The study, titled *Your Brain on ChatGPT*, determined that delegating complex cognitive work to AI can lead to "cognitive debt," where users become less engaged and retain less information, confirming that AI is not a substitute for the foundational cognitive work of brainstorming, structuring arguments, and recalling information.

The risk isn't that AI will maliciously dull our brains, but that its sheer convenience will lead us to voluntarily sidestep the essential, effortful work of thinking that builds and maintains our cognitive strength.

The Hidden Shame of AI-Assisted Writing

Beyond cognitive effort and authenticity, there is a troubling cultural tension that many clinicians and writers experience but rarely name. If AI can help draft, refine, and organize our work, then what exactly does it mean to say, *"I wrote this"?*

In practice, AI is already embedded across personal and professional writing workflows. Yet, despite its ubiquity, many remain hesitant to acknowledge its use openly. Disclosures are often softened — "just for editing" or "only for brainstorming" — as if the degree of use determines legitimacy. This pattern reflects not a failure of ethics, but a lack of shared norms.

The discomfort is not simply about ease of use. It is about identity. Writing has long been associated with individual effort, intellectual ownership, and even a certain degree of struggle. AI challenges that narrative. It introduces a form of collaboration that is immediate, iterative, and non-human, one that can feel productive in private but difficult or embarrassing to explain in public. As a result, a gap emerges between how work is actually created and how it is described to others.

This tension is compounded by a cultural attitude in which highly polished writing is sometimes viewed with suspicion. What was once a marker of clarity and skill may now be interpreted as evidence of machine assistance. In response, some writers consciously adjust their style, avoiding certain constructions or even allowing minor imperfections, to signal authenticity.

At its core, this is not a problem of technology but of culture. When expectations around AI use are unclear, individuals default to silence or defensiveness rather than transparency. The issue is not whether AI is used, but how it is used. There is a meaningful difference between augmentation, where AI supports human judgment, and substitution, where it replaces it, as discussed in the opening essay.

In medical and scientific writing, that distinction is critical. The responsibility for accuracy, interpretation, and ethical integrity remains firmly human. AI may assist in shaping the prose, but it does not bear accountability for the content.

A Case in Point

The recent controversy surrounding *Shy Girl* by Mia Ballard underscores how quickly concerns about AI-assisted writing can escalate from abstract debate to concrete consequence. Hachette Book Group halted publication and withdrew the novel from distribution after internal review, following widespread online speculation that portions of the text resembled AI-generated prose.

Readers on platforms like Goodreads and Reddit had begun dissecting passages, raising questions about authorship and originality. Whether or not Ballard herself directly used AI, the outcome is notable: a published work effectively erased from the marketplace and a writer's reputation placed under intense scrutiny. It represents one of the first high-profile instances in which AI-related concerns have led to a tangible professional penalty in publishing.

This episode may prove to be a turning point. The boundary between acceptable assistance and unacceptable substitution remains poorly defined, yet enforcement has begun nonetheless. Ballard's attribution of responsibility to a collaborator further complicates the issue, highlighting how diffuse authorship has become in an era of AI tools, ghostwriters, and hybrid work arrangements.

For now, the lesson is less about where the line definitively lies and more about how unforgiving the consequences may be when that line is perceived to have been crossed. As publishers, professional organizations, and authors attempt to establish norms, such as emerging labeling initiatives to distinguish human-authored work, cases like this are likely to multiply. The debate over AI and writing is no longer theoretical; it is disciplinary, reputational, and, increasingly, career-defining.

The Challenge: Transparent Use

The emerging challenge, then, is not to eliminate AI from writing, but to accept and normalize thoughtful, transparent use. As with prior technological shifts, the goal is to integrate new tools without disregarding the standards that define the work. We should remember that writing in any capacity remains hard work — intellectual, iterative, and often uncomfortable. As Robert A. Heinlein wryly observed, "Writing is not necessarily something to be ashamed of, but do it in private and wash your hands afterwards."

The point endures: The act of writing has always carried a certain vulnerability and resistance. AI may ease parts of the process, but it does not eliminate the responsibility or the effort required to think clearly, judge wisely, and say something worth reading. So, when someone asks, "Why should I bother to read what nobody bothered to write?", the polite response is that the measure of writing is not how it was assisted, but whether it reflects careful thought, human judgment, and something genuinely worth saying.

Several major CEOs and leaders in the publishing and media industries have openly embraced AI, though their levels of acceptance and how they use it vary. Barnes & Noble CEO James Daunt stated in a 2026 NBC News article that he has no problem stocking and selling books written by AI in stores across the country, as long as the AI authorship is transparently labeled, customers want to buy them, and they don't plagiarize other authors. Most publishing CEOs draw the line at AI being used as original authorship for contracted authors and generally support industry regulations to protect intellectual property.

Future Directions

The role of AI in medical writing is poised to grow. New systems are being designed to provide citations by default, highlight uncertainty, and integrate reporting checklists into drafting. Increasingly, AI will also support multimodal content creation, generating not only text but also graphics, audio abstracts, and short videos from the same source material.

Specialty-specific models trained on curated medical corpora may reduce factual errors, while real-time collaborative editing tools will allow authors and AI to work seamlessly within shared platforms.

Perhaps most importantly, AI will expand the personalization and accessibility of medical communication, adapting a single document into multiple versions tailored to clinicians, patients, or policymakers. This evolution will reinforce the shift in the writer's role: from sole content creator to curator, editor, and ethical steward, ensuring that every automated gain preserves trust and scientific integrity.

Conclusion

AI has matured from a convenience feature into a powerful partner in medical writing. It accelerates literature mapping, supports clear narrative structure, and broadens accessibility. But fluency does not equate to truth. The human writer remains responsible for accuracy, evidence, and interpretation.

The most effective approach is to treat AI as one would a capable assistant: Set explicit tasks, constrain its scope, demand transparency, and carefully review its work. With this disciplined, ethically informed use, AI can help medical writers produce documents that are faster to prepare, more polished in form, and more impactful in reaching their intended audiences: clinicians, patients, policymakers, and the public alike.

REFERENCE

1. Kosmyna N, Hauptmann E, Yuan YT, Situ J, Liao XH, *et al.* Your brain on ChatGPT: accumulation of cognitive debt when using an AI assistant for essay writing task. MIT Media Lab. 2025. https://arxiv.org/pdf/2506.08872.

Using AI Responsibly in Medical Writing: A Practical Checklist

Stage	Key Actions	Purpose
1. Before You Begin	• Understand basics of machine learning (ML), natural language processing (NLP), and large language models (LLMs). • Select secure, transparent tools aligned with institutional and publisher policies.	Establish foundational knowledge and ensure appropriate, compliant tool selection.
2. During the Writing Process	• Use AI for efficiency: literature scoping, outlining, drafting, style harmonization, and reference management. • Provide curated inputs (notes, selected articles) to reduce errors. • Critically review outputs: fact-check all claims and verify references.	Enhance productivity while maintaining accuracy and intellectual rigor.
3. Ethical and Legal Safeguards	• Never upload protected health information (PHI) or proprietary data to public platforms. • Treat AI as a tool, not an author; disclose use per guidelines. • Run plagiarism/similarity checks to ensure originality.	Protect confidentiality, ensure ethical authorship, and maintain academic integrity.
4. After Drafting	• Confirm compliance with reporting standards (CONSORT, PRISMA, STROBE, CARE) and journal formatting. • Ensure clarity for the intended audience (clinicians, patients, policymakers, public). • Document workflow (tools, versions, purposes) for transparency.	Ensure completeness, readability, and transparency prior to submission.
5. Pressure Testing	• Neutral appraisal: Prompt AI for an unbiased review. • Devil's advocate: Identify logical gaps or unsupported claims. • Positive view: Request a solutions-oriented critique balancing support with rigor.	Strengthen arguments through structured, multi-perspective evaluation.

Essay 3.

The Promise and Peril of AI Scribes

For decades, physicians have dreamed of a simple technological solution to one of modern medicine's most corrosive burdens: documentation.

The electronic health record promised efficiency but delivered something quite different: extra burden. Physicians now spend hours each evening completing notes, clicking boxes, and reconciling fields in what has become known as "pajama time." The keyboard has often replaced eye contact. The screen has displaced the patient.

Ambient AI scribes arrived with the promise of reversing this trajectory, although, as I discuss in the subsequent essay, the gains may be more limited in specialties such as oncology and psychiatry, where nuanced conversations and complex clinical reasoning resist easy transcription.

In principle, the concept of employing AI scribes is elegant. Software listens to the conversation between doctor and patient, transcribes it, and generates a structured clinical note that the physician edits and signs. The physician can remain focused on the patient rather than the computer.

Early data suggest the benefits may be real.[1] One large implementation across more than 2.5 million encounters reported dramatic reductions in documentation time, saving physicians an estimated 15,700 hours of note-writing in a single year while improving physician satisfaction and patient interaction.

For many clinicians, the technology feels like a long-awaited reprieve. Yet as with nearly every technological advance in medicine, the early narrative is more complicated than the promotional headlines suggest.

A growing body of research suggests that while AI scribes may alleviate clerical burden, they also introduce new categories of risk, particularly in the subtle terrain where documentation and clinical reasoning intersect.

One analysis of real-world clinician feedback identified multiple types of patient safety concerns arising from AI-generated notes.[2]

These concerns included incorrect medication names and dosages, fabricated or inaccurate medical history, misattribution of statements between patient and clinician, and omissions of key discussion points about diagnoses or treatment decisions.

Even more concerning, some reports described what clinicians increasingly recognize as a familiar phenomenon in generative AI: hallucinations. The scribe occasionally inserted diagnoses, exam findings, or clinical details that had never been discussed during the encounter. Such errors are not necessarily common, but their presence is noteworthy (pun intended).

A transcription error in a grocery list is inconsequential. A transcription error in a clinical record can alter treatment decisions, billing codes, or medicolegal documentation. The technology's promise, therefore, sits alongside a fundamental clinical reality: Physicians remain responsible for every word in the chart.

Interestingly, physicians' experience with AI scribes reflects a pattern that historians of technology would recognize instantly.[3] Early adopters report both enthusiasm and unease. Qualitative interviews of physicians using ambient AI scribes reveal overwhelmingly positive reactions regarding workload and patient engagement. Many clinicians report improved eye contact, more natural conversations, and reduced cognitive strain during visits.

Yet those same interviews reveal persistent dissatisfaction with accuracy, note construction, and editing requirements. Physicians frequently report transcription mistakes, misheard words, or stylistic issues that require substantial revision before a note can be finalized. The result is an ironic paradox: The technology designed to eliminate documentation burden sometimes shifts that burden into a different form: editing rather than writing (see Essay 16).

This pattern is not unique to AI scribes. It reflects a broader truth about early technological adoption in medicine. The first generation of any new tool tends to produce two reactions simultaneously: optimism and overconfidence.

Optimism is understandable. Physicians who have struggled for years with inefficient documentation systems are understandably eager for anything that restores time and attention to patient care.

The possibility of reclaiming the human side of medicine is deeply appealing.

Overconfidence, however, can be more subtle. When a technology performs well most of the time, users may begin to trust it more than they should. Automation bias — the human tendency to defer to machine-generated outputs — has been documented across multiple domains of clinical decision support.[4]

The same risk applies to documentation systems. If an AI-generated note appears polished and complete, the temptation is to skim rather than scrutinize. That temptation may be particularly strong at the end of a long clinic day.

But a chart is not merely a record of a conversation. It is a clinical artifact that influences downstream care. Consultants read it, nurses rely on it, pharmacists verify medications through it, and lawyers examine it when outcomes are questioned. In other words, the note is not just a summary. It is infrastructure.

There is also a significant concern that goes beyond accuracy. Documentation has historically been part of the thinking process itself. As one *JAMA* commentary observed, dictation once forced physicians to organize their thoughts aloud — to transform scattered observations into a coherent narrative of clinical reasoning.[5] In that sense, the consult note was not merely documentation but a cognitive pause in which understanding took shape. As AI-generated documentation becomes more automated, some of that reflective work may no longer occur.

The implications extend beyond the exam room. Consider this personal experience that occurred about a half-hour into a recent virtual work meeting, conducted on Microsoft Teams with an ambient AI scribe operating silently in the background. The limits of passive listening became suddenly apparent.

A colleague was participating in the meeting while driving. He began, "The company has developed their own policy for that. They combined it with the state's Medicaid policy. We thought it was a great idea, and so we went ahead and adopted it, and oh ****, I've got a ****** flat tire. Oh, I'm sorry, just swearing while driving. Oh my God, anyway. Um."

I responded instinctively: "Be safe. Be safe. If you have to pull over — if you have to leave us and pull over — do so."

Somewhere in the background, the ambient scribe was listening — faithfully, indiscriminately, unemotionally. One can only imagine the draft summary: a seamless paragraph integrating Medicaid policy, corporate governance, and a punctuated roadside emergency. The software cannot distinguish between strategic discussion and startled profanity. It captures everything. Context, relevance, and judgment remain human responsibilities.

The anecdote is comical, but the lesson is serious. AI excels at transcription and pattern recognition. It does not reliably determine what matters. It does not recognize urgency (fortunately, no harm came to my colleague).

This is where the conversation about AI scribes must mature. The question is not whether the technology is useful. By most accounts, it clearly is. Reducing physician documentation burden is a worthy goal, and restoring face-to-face attention between doctors and patients may be one of the most meaningful improvements digital health can deliver.

But without human intervention, in this instance, my administrative assistant, who smoothed over the incident in the final, edited meeting minutes, the record would have remained technically accurate yet contextually misleading, capturing the words but not the intent, and preserving a version of events that obscured more than it clarified.

This speaks to the more important question of how we integrate these tools effectively. That integration requires humility about the limits of current systems. It requires rigorous monitoring for errors that may emerge only after widespread deployment. It requires thoughtful workflow design so that physicians remain active editors rather than passive signers of machine-generated notes. Most importantly, it requires preserving a core principle of medical professionalism: responsibility cannot be automated.

Technology can assist. It can augment. It can streamline. But the final act of clinical documentation — the moment when the note becomes part of the patient's permanent medical record — remains a human responsibility. This is true in virtually all contexts.

For example, research examining the use of large language models to review health insurance plan documents for compliance with the Mental Health Parity and Addiction Equity Act found that while AI could analyze hundreds of pages of policy language in seconds, its accuracy was only about 49%, meaning human regulators still had to review the results to remove spurious findings and confirm real violations.[6]

The lesson is familiar. AI can dramatically accelerate the search for problems, but it cannot yet reliably determine which problems are real. Human judgment remains the final safeguard. Medicine is no different. AI may draft the note, but the physician must still read it, correct it, and stand behind it.

What is ultimately at stake may not be documentation efficiency but something more subtle: the preservation of clinical reasoning itself. Writing or dictating a note has historically forced physicians to pause, organize scattered observations, and commit to an interpretation of the case. It is a moment when uncertainty is shaped into narrative, and the clinician's thinking becomes visible. When that narrative arrives preassembled by an algorithm, the temptation is to accept it rather than construct it.

The danger is not that AI will write the note poorly, but that physicians may gradually relinquish the cognitive work the note once required. The chart may become more polished, yet the thinking behind it may be thinner. In the long run, the greatest risk of automated documentation may not be what the machine adds to the record, but what the clinician no longer has to think through before signing it.

REFERENCES

1. Tierney AA, Gayre G, Hoberman B, Mattern B, Ballesca M, *et al.* Ambient artificial intelligence scribes: learnings after 1 year and over 2.5 million uses. *NEJM Catal Innov Care Deliv.* 2025;6(5). https://catalyst.nejm.org/doi/full/10.1056/CAT.25.0040.
2. Dai J, Huang A, Nasarallah C, Croci R, Soleimani H, *et al.* Patient safety risks from AI scribes: signals from end-user feedback. December 2025. arXiv:2512.04118. https://doi.org/10.48550/arXiv.2512.04118.
3. Shah SJ, Crowell T, Jeong Y, Devon-Sand A, Smith M, Yang B, *et al.* Physician perspectives on ambient AI scribes. *JAMA Netw Open.* 2025;8(3):e241904. https://doi.org/10.1001/jamanetworkopen.2025.1904.

4. Goddard K, Roudsari A, Wyatt JC. Automation bias: a systematic review of frequency, effect mediators, and mitigators. *J Am Med Inform Assoc.* 2011;19(1):121–127. https://doi.org/10.1136/amiajnl-2011-000089.
5. Chin-Yee B. The death of the consult note. *JAMA*. 2026;335(10):854–855. doi:10.1001/jama.2025.26848.
6. Counts NZ. Large language models for efficient mental health parity oversight. *Psychiatr Serv*. 2026;77(4). https://doi.org/10.1176/appi.ps.20250178.

Essay 4.

When AI Writes the Therapy Note, the Patient's Story Can Disappear

Imagine a patient who spends most of a therapy session talking about a single memory. He describes sitting in his car after visiting his mother in a nursing home, shaken and unable to start the engine. He sits there for nearly 20 minutes, staring at the steering wheel and wondering when the roles had reversed — when he had become the parent and she the child.

Nothing dramatic happens in the session. No real breakthrough. No targeted intervention. But the moment is clinically significant. It reveals a developmental turning point — from seeing parents as authority figures to recognizing them as aging, imperfect individuals — along with the complex emotions that accompany that realization: grief, guilt, sadness, and disillusionment.

If an AI-generated progress note had summarized the session, it might have read something like this: "Patient reports situational sadness related to family stressors. Supportive therapy provided. Coping strategies reviewed."

The note would be technically correct, but the story — the heart of the encounter — would have disappeared.

AI is rapidly entering psychotherapy practices, promising relief from one of the profession's most tedious burdens: documentation. Many systems now record therapy sessions, transcribe them, and automatically generate progress notes. The pitch is simple: Let the algorithm write the note so the therapist can focus on the patient.

But the reality emerging from clinicians and researchers suggests something more problematic.[1] When AI writes the therapy note, efficiency may increase, but meaning may be stripped away.

Efficiency versus Meaning

AI-assisted documentation tools are spreading quickly across behavioral health platforms. They record sessions, produce transcripts, and convert them into structured notes aligned with treatment plans and diagnostic codes. In theory, this allows therapists to remain more present during the session.

In practice, however, the outputs often compress the reality of human experience into standardized templates. Clinicians reviewing AI-generated notes frequently report that the documentation is technically accurate yet narratively hollow. Summaries capture symptoms and interventions but fail to convey the patient's lived experience. The result can feel less like a clinical narrative and more like an administrative artifact.

This should not surprise us. Large language models are trained to detect patterns in text, not meaning in suffering. Psychotherapy depends on nuance — the hesitation in a voice, the contradictions inside a sentence, the emotional weight of a memory that surfaces unexpectedly. These moments shape clinical understanding, yet they are difficult to translate into automated summaries.

When the Algorithm Invents the Story

Even more troubling are reports of AI-generated notes inserting details that never occurred in the session, not unlike the well-documented phenomenon of inaccuracies creeping into medical charts, as mentioned in the previous essay. Therapists have described documentation that referenced suicidal ideation, substance abuse, or past trauma that the patient never mentioned. In one reported case, a note falsely documented a history of childhood sexual abuse.[2]

Such errors are not merely clerical. Once entered into a medical record, they can shape clinical impressions, influence treatment decisions, and surface in legal proceedings. AI hallucinations (the generation of plausible but false information) are a known feature of large language models. In psychotherapy documentation, however, these hallucinations carry consequences far beyond an incorrect sentence in a report. They can distort the patient's narrative and bury the truth, or create a totally false impression.

Psychotherapy Is Not Just Data

The interest in AI tools in mental health care is understandable. Mental health systems worldwide face severe workforce shortages and rising demand for services. Digital technologies, including AI chatbots and automated support tools, may help expand access to psychological care.

Some studies suggest AI-driven systems can reduce anxiety and provide immediate emotional support when therapists are unavailable.[3] But traditional psychotherapy consistently produces greater improvements in symptoms, likely because human clinicians provide emotional depth and adaptive responsiveness that AI systems cannot replicate.

AI may be able to summarize therapy, but it cannot conduct it. Psychotherapy depends on relational attunement: the subtle interplay between therapist and patient through which meaning emerges over time. An algorithm can process words. It cannot perceive silence and respond to it.

In the 2025 French mystery thriller *A Private Life*, the psychiatrist, Dr. Lilian Steiner (played by Jodie Foster), begins the film meticulously recording her sessions on MiniDiscs, documenting every encounter. But by the end of the film, she abandons the recorder entirely, rebuilding her practice around something simpler and far more difficult: listening. The change reflects a realization familiar to many clinicians, that what matters most in therapy is not the transcript of what was said, but the human presence required to hear what was meant.

The Narrative Function of the Therapy Note

Historically, psychotherapy notes served two purposes. They documented clinical care. They also helped therapists think, just as they did medical consultants, as previously discussed. Writing a note forces the clinician to reconstruct the session: What was important? What changed? What remained unresolved? Documentation itself is part of the reflective process.

When AI generates the note, that reflective step might not occur. The therapist reviews the summary, corrects a few errors, and signs the note. The act of writing — of re-entering the patient's narrative — is replaced by editing. Efficiency improves. Reflection diminishes. Over time, that shift may subtly change how clinicians process psychotherapy itself, from an interpretive, meaning-making exercise into a task of verification and correction.

The Story Is the Treatment

AI will almost certainly remain part of the future of mental health care. Used wisely, it may help manage administrative burdens, identify patterns in behavior, and extend support between sessions. But these systems must remain tools. The therapist must remain responsible not only for the accuracy of the clinical record, but for preserving the patient's story.

Psychotherapy is not simply a collection of symptoms, interventions, and billing codes. It is a narrative process in which patients reconstruct their lives through conversation. In *Narrative Medicine in the Age of Uncertainty*, I argue that when systems strain, as they increasingly do in modern healthcare, stories steady us.[4] They restore the conversations that speed, bureaucracy, and technology threaten to eliminate.

AI-generated notes risk doing precisely that: removing the story in the name of efficiency. If we allow that to happen, psychotherapy documentation may become technically perfect yet clinically muted. And in a field where the story guides the treatment, losing the story means losing the soul of the work itself.

REFERENCES

1. Cecil J, Schaffernak I, Evangelou D, Lermer E, Gaube S, Klein AK. Navigating the complexity of AI adoption in psychotherapy by identifying key facilitators and barriers. *npj Mental Health Res*. 2026;5(17). https://doi.org/10.1038/s44184-026-00199-1.
2. Pinder J. Therapy notes by AI create false narratives, therapists say. ClearHealthCosts. March 13, 2025. https://clearhealthcosts.com/blog/2025/03/therapy-notes-by-ai-create-false-narratives-therapists-say/.
3. Spytska L. The use of artificial intelligence in psychotherapy: development of intelligent therapeutic systems. *BMC Psychol*. 2025;13(1):175. https://doi.org/10.1186/s40359-025-02491-9.
4. Lazarus A. *Narrative Medicine in the Age of Uncertainty*. Self-published. 2026.

Essay 5.

Why the Silence? Reflections on the Vanishing Physician Commentariat

A colleague recently asked me a simple question that turned out to be anything but simple.

John Joseph Pack, MD, the retired internist who hosts the thoughtful online publication *GrandRoundsMD*, told me that readership analytics for the site are strong. Physicians are clearly reading the essays. They are opening the articles, spending time with them, and returning to the website. Yet almost no one is commenting.

I've observed this on other websites geared toward physicians: thoughtful essays and opinion pieces drawing no comments. Why is this the case, Dr. Pack wondered, when the very purpose of his publication is dialogue?

It is a perplexing phenomenon, especially given the aspirations of the site itself. *GrandRoundsMD* was created to restore humanity to the practice of medicine, to create a space where physicians share stories that heal, where wisdom and ethics can be discussed alongside science, and where the profession might reconnect with its deeper sense of purpose. The mission statement reads less like a corporate prospectus than a manifesto for reclaiming medicine's intellectual and moral center.

And yet the comment section beneath many articles sits quietly, like an empty conference room after a meeting that never quite started.

The silence is striking because physicians have never lacked opinions. If anything, we are famous for them. Walk into any hospital lounge or conference corridor, and you will hear vigorous debate about everything from clinical guidelines to health policy to the latest administrative directive. Doctors argue, analyze, and reflect. It is part of the intellectual culture of the profession.

But the venue has changed. Increasingly, it seems that physicians prefer to read in silence.

Part of this practice may simply reflect the broader cultural migration of discourse. Conversations that once took place in website comment sections have moved to social media platforms where engagement is more visible, immediate, and algorithmically multiplied. A comment on LinkedIn may reach thousands of readers. A comment on a niche website may reach only a handful. In a profession already pressed for time, the incentive structure is important.

Yet that explanation feels incomplete. I suspect something deeper is at work, something that has been gradually reshaping how physicians interact with one another in public spaces.

Several years ago, I wrote an editorial reflecting on the darker side of online physician discourse.[1] A very small number of commenters, I noted, had managed to create a toxic atmosphere on some medical websites, engaging in personal attacks and unprofessional exchanges that discouraged participation. Burnout and frustration within the profession seemed to fuel these interactions, turning what should have been constructive dialogue into incivility.

The result was predictable. Many physicians simply disengaged. The loudest voices remained, while the more reflective ones stepped away.

Anyone who has moderated online discussions, as I did for *Doximity* at one time, recognizes this dynamic. The majority of readers — often attentive, experienced clinicians — prefer not to enter a conversation that might quickly devolve into acrimony. Even when moderators intervene, the damage is often already done. Once a space acquires a reputation for hostility, the silent majority retreats as a form of self-preservation.

There is another factor as well: fatigue. Modern physicians live within an environment saturated with commentary. Email alerts, newsletters, journal updates, social media feeds, and policy announcements compete constantly for attention. Reading itself has become a form of triage. One scans, absorbs, reflects, and moves on to the next demand.

Commenting requires something additional: emotional and

intellectual energy. For many clinicians already experiencing administrative burdens, documentation demands, and the psychological weight of patient care, that extra step may simply feel like too much. So, they read. They think. But they do not respond.

Ironically, this silent readership may represent a kind of respect. When physicians encounter writing that resonates, writing that captures something true about their professional lives, they often internalize it rather than debate it publicly. The reflection continues privately, in the car ride home, during a morning walk, or in a quiet moment between patients.

Narrative medicine has always understood this phenomenon. Stories do not always provoke an immediate response. Sometimes they work slowly, settling into the reader's consciousness and reshaping how experiences are interpreted. The absence of comments does not necessarily mean the absence of impact. Still, the quiet is unsettling.

Medicine today faces enormous structural pressures: consolidation, corporatization, technological acceleration, and the loss of professional autonomy. Physicians often feel, as Dr. Pack describes in his mission statement, like a ship without a rudder: propelled forward by forces we did not choose and cannot easily control. In such a moment, however, professional dialogue is important because it restores a measure of agency, allowing clinicians to interpret, question, and shape the powers that otherwise seem to direct them.

The original spirit of medical "grand rounds" was not merely educational; it was communal. Physicians gathered to discuss cases, share insights, challenge assumptions, and learn collectively. The process was inherently interactive. Questions were asked. Perspectives were offered. Knowledge evolved through conversation.

A publication like *GrandRoundsMD* attempts to recreate that ethos in digital form. But digital grand rounds require participants who are willing to speak.

The challenge, then, is not merely technological. It is also cultural. Physicians must rediscover a sense of collective voice, not only through essays and articles, but through respectful, collegial exchange. Disagreement should be expected. Medicine advances through debate. But that debate must be grounded in professionalism and mutual respect. Otherwise, silence will continue to dominate.

There is a paradox here worth acknowledging. Physicians frequently lament the loss of influence within healthcare systems increasingly governed by corporate priorities and financial dashboards. Yet influence requires participation. A profession that withdraws from public dialogue risks further marginalization.

Commenting on an essay may seem like a small act. In reality, it represents something larger: engagement in the ongoing conversation about what medicine is and what it should become.

Perhaps the solution begins modestly. A brief reflection beneath an article. A respectful question. A perspective drawn from clinical experience. The digital equivalent of raising one's hand during grand rounds. Not every comment will be profound. Not every debate will change the profession. But the act of speaking counts.

Dr. Pack's vision for *GrandRoundsMD* is, in many ways, a hopeful one. He imagines a space where physicians reconnect with one another intellectually and ethically, where stories illuminate the human side of care, and where the profession begins once again to chart its own course.

That kind of community cannot be built by analytics alone. It requires voices. The essays may start the conversation. But it is the comments that keep it alive.

REFERENCE

1. Lazarus A. The dos and don'ts of posting comments on medical websites. *J Medical Pract Manag*. February 8, 2022. https://www.physicianleaders.org/articles/dos-donts-posting-comments-medical-websites.

Essay 6.

When Is a Joke Not a Joke? Medicine, Social Media, and the Return of the Physician Commentariat

In the previous essay, I lamented the disappearance of the physician commentariat. Doctors, I said, had grown quiet in public debates about medicine. Burnout, institutional constraints, and professional risk had pushed many physicians into silence. Yet the reaction to a recent viral social media post by a medical student at Mayo Clinic suggests the physician commentariat has not vanished; it has migrated.

Today, medical discourse unfolds not primarily in journals or conference halls, but on Instagram, X, TikTok, LinkedIn, Bluesky, and comment threads beneath viral posts. These are arenas where professional norms collide with internet culture, where context collapses, and where a joke can ignite a profession-wide argument within hours and appear on national television that evening.

The controversy surrounding the Mayo Clinic medical student illustrates how complicated this new landscape has become, especially when considering a student labeled as a "TikTok star" with 360,000 followers.

The Joke That Launched a Thousand Comments

The student's post shows him handing a woman a copy of the *Diagnostic and Statistical Manual of Mental Disorders (DSM-5)* while implying that the book was "written for her." The woman, it later emerged, was his sister. The tone was presented as sibling banter.

To some viewers, the joke was harmless. Many comments echoed the sentiment:

"It's not that deep."

"Typical sibling humor."

"People are too sensitive."

To others, particularly physicians in women's health, the post represented something far more ominous.

An OB/GYN physician who posts under the name "gynogirl" argued that the joke echoed a long and damaging tradition in medicine: the dismissal of women's physical symptoms as psychological or "hysterical." She pointed to conditions such as endometriosis, vulvodynia, autoimmune disease, and heart disease — conditions in which women historically experienced delayed diagnosis or misattribution of symptoms.

In that interpretation, the joke was not merely humor. It was a cultural echo of one of medicine's great failures: the minimization of women's symptoms and the tendency to recast physical suffering as psychological distress. And that difference — between a joke heard as harmless and a joke heard as historical reenactment — is precisely where the debate exploded.

"Hysteria" Lingers

To understand the intensity of the response, one must understand the history. For centuries, the diagnosis of hysteria functioned as a medical catch-all for symptoms that physicians could not explain (or chose not to investigate) and instead attributed them to emotional or nervous causes. The term derives from the Greek *hystera*, meaning uterus. In ancient medicine, hysteria was linked to the theory of the "wandering womb," the belief that the uterus could migrate within the body and produce physical and psychological symptoms.

Physicians later abandoned the literal notion of uterine wandering, as well as the term "hysteria" (though not entirely). Still, the association between women's reproductive organs and presumed emotional instability has persisted, and the underlying dynamic dismissing unexplained symptoms as psychological remains a topic of ongoing debate. Studies continue to show that women with certain conditions wait longer for diagnosis and treatment, particularly in cardiology and specialties dealing with autoimmune diseases.

So, when a joke summons a psychiatric manual in response to a woman's behavior, some clinicians do not hear a casual gag. They hear a centuries-old reflex. That is why the word "hysteria," even when not explicitly used, can ignite strong reactions in medical spaces.

But Is It Gaslighting?

Some critics would go further, calling the med student's video an example of medical gaslighting. Medical gaslighting refers to the invalidation of a patient's genuine symptoms or concerns by a healthcare professional, leading the patient to doubt their own perceptions or reality. The term "gaslighting" originates from the 1938 play *Gas Light* (and its 1940 and 1944 film adaptations), in which a husband manipulates environmental cues (notably dimming gas lights) and denies it, causing his wife to doubt her sanity.

Calling the video "gaslighting" stretches the concept, however. When every offensive or tone-deaf remark becomes gaslighting, the term loses analytical precision. But this does not mean the criticism itself is illegitimate. It simply means we should describe the problem accurately. What we are witnessing is not gaslighting. It is symbolic signaling: a joke that inadvertently touches a sensitive cultural nerve within medicine.

Humor, Professionalism, and Context Collapse

Humor inside medicine has always existed. Medical students joke about exam stress. Residents joke about call schedules. Physicians trade dark humor about the emotional toll of practice. Gallows humor has long been a coping mechanism, perhaps best exemplified by Samuel Shem's 1978 novel *The House of God*, in which interns at a fictional Boston teaching hospital use irreverent, often biting humor and terms like "GOMER" ("Get Out of My Emergency Room") to distance themselves from the suffering, hierarchy, and distress of internship. But social media has altered the environment in which humor operates.

A joke shared among friends is not the same as a joke posted to a platform where millions of strangers, including patients, can see it. This phenomenon is known as *context collapse*. The audience becomes unknowable. What was intended as personal humor becomes public messaging. For physicians and trainees, this move can have serious consequences.

Medicine is a profession grounded in trust. Patients routinely disclose their most vulnerable experiences: physical, psychological, and social. Even the appearance of dismissiveness toward those experiences can undermine confidence. Thus, the central question is not whether the student meant harm. It is whether physicians should consider how their humor appears when broadcast to a public audience that includes patients.

Should Mayo Clinic Discipline the Student?

Disciplinary action lies at the center of the controversy. Some commenters demanded expulsion from medical school. Others argued that disciplining a student for a joke would represent an overreach of institutional authority. Legally and ethically, the situation falls into a gray zone.

Private institutions, including medical schools, generally retain broad authority to regulate conduct that affects their professional environment or public reputation. Most medical schools maintain professionalism codes that apply not only to clinical settings but also to online behavior. This authority is not unlimited, but it is vested and material.

The key distinction is that medical training is not merely an educational program. It is preparation for a licensed profession entrusted with public welfare. The same logic that governs bedside professionalism often extends to digital spaces. However, professional discipline should distinguish between malicious misconduct and immature judgment. Not every lapse requires career-ending consequences. Medicine has long believed in education, mentorship, and remediation. Those principles should apply here as well.

The medical student deleted his TikTok and Instagram accounts. It is unknown whether Mayo pressured him to do it or whether the sheer amount of backlash resulted in a voluntary decision to remove his accounts. It's quite possible that continuing his online presence, even if permitted by Mayo and toned down, could have unwanted repercussions for a residency position. As events unfolded, however, the question of future residency prospects became irrelevant, as the student was reportedly expelled from medical school — at least according to online accounts.

The Curious Case of "Gynogirl"

The controversy also raises another interesting question. If language and symbolism matter, what about the critic's own online identity? The physician who started the controversy posts under the moniker "gynogirl."

Some observers have asked whether such branding is itself potentially problematic. Does it trivialize professional identity? Does it reinforce gender labeling in a specialty that already has its share of gender politics?

These questions are not accusations. They simply highlight a broader reality of social media: everyone participating in online discourse brings their own framing, language, and branding choices. In the internet age, criticism rarely travels in one direction.

Why Physicians Fight So Fiercely Online

The rancor in the comment threads may surprise outsiders. Why would physicians, members of a profession devoted to healing, engage in such combative exchanges? Several forces are at work.

First, medicine today exists under intense scrutiny. Social media broadcasts every controversy, and physicians often feel compelled to defend their profession or their patients.

Second, professional identity in medicine has become increasingly fragile. Burnout, administrative pressures, and systemic changes have left many physicians feeling that the values of the profession are under threat. When controversies arise, they become symbolic battlegrounds for deeper anxieties about the future of medicine.

Third, online platforms reward outrage. Algorithms elevate emotionally charged content because it generates engagement, and engagement sometimes turns into dollars and cents, depending on the platform. What begins as disagreement quickly escalates into moral confrontation.

The Commentariat Has Not Vanished

Which brings us back to the original question: Has the physician commentariat really disappeared? Clearly not. Physicians are speaking more than ever. But they are speaking in different venues: Instagram threads instead of journal editorials, TikTok videos instead of conference panels.

The style has changed as well. Traditional medical commentary emphasized careful reasoning, evidence, and moderation. Social media commentary favors speed, emotion, and visibility.

Both forms have value. Both have risks. But the migration of professional discourse into algorithm-driven spaces fundamentally alters how and when medical debates unfold.

AI Amplification

This transformation connects directly to a broader theme: the increasing role of AI-mediated systems in shaping professional communication (discussed in the next essay). Social media platforms are not neutral arenas. Their algorithms decide which posts gain visibility and which disappear. Engagement metrics — "likes," shares, and comments — drive amplification.

In effect, machine-learning systems are already curating medical discourse. A joke that might once have circulated among a few friends can now reach millions because an algorithm detects that it generates emotional responses.

The controversy surrounding the Mayo student did not spread solely because of human attention. It spread because AI-driven recommendation engines recognized the post as high-engagement content. This dynamic will only intensify. As generative AI begins producing medical commentary, summarizing debates, and recommending content to clinicians and patients alike, the boundaries between professional discourse and algorithmic intensification will blur even further.

The commentariat is no longer entirely human.

The Deeper Lesson

The real lesson of this episode is not that humor must disappear from medicine, nor that every offensive remark requires understanding its historical origins or meting out institutional punishment. The lesson is simpler.

Medicine now operates in an environment where professional identity, public trust, and algorithmic augmentation intersect. A joke can become a symbol. A comment thread can become a national debate. And a medical student's Instagram post can trigger a profession-wide argument about history, gender, professionalism, and speech.

The physician commentariat has not vanished. It has been redistributed across platforms governed partly by machines. In the age of AI, the conversation about medicine — its ethics, its humor, its blind spots — will increasingly occur in spaces where algorithms determine what rises to the surface. That reality may be difficult to digest. But it is now part of practicing medicine.

Essay 7.

The Compression of Language by AI

Language has always evolved. Words shorten, meanings vary, and communication adapts to the technologies of the day. The telegraph compressed sentences into coded bursts. Text messaging gave us abbreviations and emojis. Social media turned thoughts into hashtags.

Now artificial intelligence may be accelerating a different kind of linguistic evolution, one that compresses not only words, but the very structure of communication. It is subtle at first. A character limit here. A summarization tool there. A medical progress note automatically condensed by an AI scribe. Over time, however, the cumulative effect begins to resemble a cultural shift toward compressed language: shorter, flatter, more standardized expressions of thought. The phenomenon appears to be emerging across medicine and society.

From Narrative to Bullet Points

Consider the modern clinical note. Not long ago, physicians often wrote narrative descriptions of patient encounters. The prose could be uneven (sometimes lofty, sometimes hurried), but it reflected the clinician's reasoning and the patient's story.

Electronic health records changed that dynamic. Templates and dropdown checkboxes replaced paragraphs. Notes became structured, standardized, and measurable.

Now, as described in Essay 3, AI scribes promise to streamline documentation even further. They listen to clinical conversations, generate summaries, and produce concise notes optimized for billing, coding, and efficiency.

The intention is good. Physicians spend far too many hours documenting care. Yet the linguistic consequence is clear: The patient's narrative becomes compressed into digestible fragments. Where once there might have been a paragraph describing uncertainty, emotion, or diagnostic reasoning, there is now a summary line. In internal medicine, it might read as:

"Patient reports intermittent chest discomfort; workup negative to date. Symptoms likely stress-related. Reassurance provided."

— or, in the compressed cadence of the modern note:

"Chest pain — noncardiac suspected. Labs WNL. Plan: reassurance, follow-up PRN."

Both lines are efficient. Both are technically correct. Yet somewhere between the patient's story and the final entry in the chart, the narrative — hesitation, doubt, the lived experience of illness — has been compressed into a few clinically acceptable words or abbreviations.

This trend extends beyond clinical documentation. AI systems increasingly summarize emails, messages, and documents into bullet points. Emotionally complex exchanges can be reduced to robotic summaries, sometimes stripping away nuance or humor entirely. Efficiency improves while meaning loses its texture.

AI's Influence on Language

Artificial intelligence does not merely compress language; it may also standardize it. Large language models generate responses by predicting the most statistically probable word sequences. Over time, this process favors common phrasing and mainstream vocabulary.

Researchers studying podcasts and conversational speech have already observed what they call "lexical seepage." Words favored by AI systems, terms like *delve*, *robust*, *profound, nuance (or nuanced)*, tend to appear with disproportionately high frequency in AI-generated text, seeping into everyday conversation and contributing to a recognizable stylistic writing fingerprint.

AI has been criticized for overuse of em dashes, creating a stylistic "tell," especially in longer works where pattern recognition (a phenomenon discussed throughout this book) makes the prose feel machine-shaped rather than author-shaped.

Similarly, writing assistants such as Grammarly or automated editing tools encourage users toward standardized constructions. Writers adapt to these suggestions, producing polished but increasingly homogeneous language styles. The result is a paradox: language becomes clearer, but less distinctive.

All of this exposure leads to imitation, and repetition leads to normalization. Eventually, the machine's linguistic habits find their way into human speech and prose. Whether this is "seepage" or simply the next phase of linguistic evolution depends on one's stance.

Language has always absorbed the dominant communicative technology of the era: the printing press, telegraph, and email. AI may simply be the newest dialect coach.

The Platform Effect

Technology platforms also shape how we communicate. Social media systems impose structural constraints such as character limits, post lengths, and algorithmic preferences that reward brevity and immediacy.

On X, posts historically fit within 280 characters. Instagram captions compete with scrolling attention spans. Hashtags condense complex ideas into searchable tags: #MedTwitter, #HealthPolicy, #AIinMedicine.

Online usernames themselves are compressed identities — handles rather than names, fragments rather than biographies. Even professional discourse increasingly conforms to these constraints. Many major medical platforms encourage essays of roughly the same length: around 800 to 1,000 words. That range is not arbitrary. It fits the attention economy of digital reading, where readers skim, editors optimize for engagement, algorithms reward completion, and compression becomes a design principle.

Narrative Medicine Meets the Word Limit

In narrative medicine, however, compression presents a challenge. Stories resist truncation. A patient's illness narrative rarely fits neatly into 1,000 words. Clinical insight often emerges in the details — an offhand remark, a remembered image, a hesitation in speech.

In my narrative medicine course, weekly writing assignments were typically limited to 800 words. The constraint was pedagogically useful: it forced students to identify the heart of a story, which could be read aloud and discussed in small groups. But shortened stories also imposed a boundary. What if the story required more space?

The same tension appears in medical publishing. Platforms such as *KevinMD*, *MedPage Today*, *Doximity*, and *Doctors on Social Media (SoMeDocs)* — my go-to websites for publishing essays and op-eds — generally favor a similar length. The format is well-suited to online readership, but it clearly shapes the kind of writing that appears there. Essays expand or contract to fit the container. Over time, writers internalize the limit.

Thinking Like a Machine

Generative AI introduces another dynamic: prompt-oriented thinking. Instead of composing ideas organically, we increasingly ask machines to summarize, condense, or rewrite our thoughts. The mental process shifts from crafting language to instructing a system how to generate it (refer to Essays 2 and 14).

Some scholars worry that this outsourcing of communication could lead to a form of linguistic atrophy. When machines summarize, tone-shift, and organize our thoughts for us, the human process of grappling with language — the struggle that produces clarity and insight — may diminish. Compression becomes not only a technological feature but a cognitive habit. We learn to speak in prompts.

A LinkedIn post captures this sentiment and perhaps a touch of overstatement. It proclaims that, with the right prompts, AI systems like Claude can "research like a Stanford PhD student," scanning dozens of papers at once, extracting themes, identifying contradictions, and mapping gaps in the literature. Research, once described as a marathon of reading and note-taking, is reframed as a process of orchestration: deploy the right prompts, and insight emerges in minutes. The advantage is no longer how much one reads, but how efficiently one can direct the machine to synthesize what matters.

The response was equally revealing and far more cautionary. One commenter pushed back, arguing that this viewpoint overlooks the most essential part of scholarship: the slow, effortful process of learning what questions to ask in the first place. It is through reading, often slow, inefficient, and frustrating, that one learns to distinguish signal from noise, to recognize the shape of a good argument, and to appreciate the many possible interpretations of the same data.

When that process is abbreviated, something more than time is saved. Something formative may be lost. The concern is not simply error, but homogenization: if many users rely on the same prompts to generate the same synthesized outputs, originality may diminish, and intellectual diversity may narrow.

Both perspectives contain truth. AI can indeed accelerate synthesis and reveal connections that might otherwise remain hidden. But the capacity to prompt effectively presupposes a prior capacity to think deeply about the material. Without that foundation, prompt-oriented thinking risks becoming an illusion of understanding — structured, fluent, and efficient, yet unmoored from the slower cognitive work that gives knowledge its depth and durability.

In addition, because AI models rely on statistical patterns drawn from massive data sets, they tend to produce mainstream or widely represented perspectives. Over time, this tendency may further narrow the diversity of ideas and narratives people encounter. If everyone receives similarly phrased answers, reads similarly structured summaries, and internalizes the same linguistic patterns, communication may converge toward a smaller set of expressions. Language may become efficient, but it also becomes predictable.

Nandini Bhattacharya, creative writing instructor at Texas A&M University, questioned, "What will happen to human originality and singularly when AI writes the same paper for everyone who posts the same prompts? AI is NOT your friend, unless you don't mind if the future is for robots and cognitively diminished humans."

The Irony of the Long Essay

These concerns partly explain why my use of AI is selective and limited primarily to language refinement rather than creation, and why many essays in this book are longer than the typical online op-ed. Editors often prefer shorter pieces. Readers expect them. Algorithms reward them.

But some ideas refuse to shrink or conform to predetermined limits. The transformation of medicine by artificial intelligence, including its ethical dilemmas, linguistic consequences, and cultural implications, rarely fits neatly within 800 to 1000 words.

Ironically, that is precisely why the compression of language deserves attention. When communication becomes optimized for speed and brevity, complexity risks becoming collateral damage.

Narrative medicine reminds us that stories are vital, but stories require space. So does thought. Which brings me to another irony of this essay. In keeping with the very trend it describes, I deliberately tried to limit it to 1,000 words, but I ran over by quite a bit.

Could I have carved out slivers to reduce the essay to editors' expectations? Of course. But in doing so, I would have performed the very act of compression the essay warns about: shaving away context and connective tissue until the argument became a cleaner summary rather than a fuller thought. Sometimes the extra words are not excess. They are the space where story lives and meaning manifests.

Section II.

Workflow, Practice, and the Clinician's Role

Essay 8.

The Algorithm in the Interview: When AI Becomes the Recruiter

What began as a promising professional exchange with a senior recruiter soon felt uncanny, like a conversation that sounded human but wasn't fully alive. The words were warm yet bloodless, polished yet mechanical. With each reply, the tone grew smoother, the phrasing more symmetrical, and the empathy increasingly synthetic. What unfolded was less a dialogue than an algorithmic echo of one.

For discretion, both the recruiter and her global pharmaceutical employer will remain unnamed. This was no fringe staffing agency, but a major corporation known for scientific rigor and humanistic branding. Yet behind that brand voice, the recruiter's emails bore the unmistakable cadence of a generative language model, likely ChatGPT or an enterprise variant.

The initial outreach was effusive and carefully flattering:

> *"Your distinguished background spanning multiple sectors reflects an exceptional blend of clinical insight, behavioral health leadership, and medical affairs strategy."*

It was followed by an invitation to discuss "alignment" with leadership opportunities, a term now as ubiquitous in AI-mediated corporate correspondence as "synergy" once was.

I replied thoughtfully, clarifying my interests in neuroscience and behavioral health leadership and noting a preference for virtual roles. The responses that followed were grammatically flawless and impeccably polite, yet curiously devoid of relational depth. Even criticism, such as a comment on my 48-page CV, was delivered in perfectly balanced prose, calibrated to signal empathy without emotion.

The final message was corporate closure distilled to its essence:

> *"We value your interest and will keep your profile under consideration as relevant opportunities progress."*

It was closure without conclusion: linguistically complete, relationally vacant.

The Linguistic Autopsy

To determine the degree of machine involvement, one needs only compare the recruiter's phrasing with standard AI-generated business language. Below is a side-by-side analysis highlighting several instances of linguistic overlap:

Recruiter's Phrases	Common ChatGPT or AI Template Equivalents	Commentary
"Your distinguished background spanning academia, managed care, and pharmaceutical leadership reflects an exceptional blend of insight and strategy."	"Your distinguished background across multiple sectors reflects an exceptional blend of experience and strategic vision."	Lexical duplication and identical syntactic rhythm suggest reuse of a standard GPT-generated compliment structure.
"At this stage, we are still in the early evaluation process for our Global Medical and Commercial Leadership initiatives."	"At this stage, we are in the early evaluation phase for our leadership opportunities."	Characteristic AI substitution of "process/phase" and "initiatives/opportunities," maintaining corporate cadence.
"We value your interest and will keep your profile under consideration as relevant opportunities progress."	"We appreciate your interest and will keep your information on file as suitable opportunities arise."	A nearly word-for-word match with ChatGPT's default closing lines in business correspondence.
"It's rare to see a professional who has led across academia, managed care, and pharmaceutical leadership with such depth."	"It's rare to find a professional whose experience spans academia, industry, and leadership with such depth."	Identical structure; ChatGPT routinely produces this "It's rare to see/find" compliment formula.
"Your resume is not doing your caliber of experience any justice."	"Your resume doesn't fully reflect the caliber of your experience and leadership."	Hallmark ChatGPT phrasing — balanced critique softened by paired nouns ("caliber" and "experience").

Each of these expressions displays language that sounds convincingly human until scrutinized for rhythm, lexical repetition, and semantic redundancy. Moreover, the emails' transitions ("Based on your background and areas of interest . . . "; "Once there is alignment . . . ") are algorithmically smooth but narratively hollow — classic signs of AI coherence optimization rather than authentic human thought.

The Verdict

Taken together, the uniform tone, syntactic symmetry, absence of imperfection, and formulaic warmth, the correspondence strongly suggested AI generation or heavy AI assistance. Most likely, the recruiter used a corporate platform integrating GPT-based tools, inserting only job titles and therapeutic areas while leaving composition to the machine.

This hybrid authorship of the recruiter as editor and the algorithm as ghostwriter may well represent the new normal in professional communication.

The Broader Implications

For senior physicians transitioning into industry, such exchanges expose a sad reality: increasingly, we are speaking with code, not colleagues. An AI-assisted recruiter does not forget credentials or lose interest, but it also does not truly see the candidate. It recognizes keywords like "neuroscience," "leadership," and "behavioral health," but not character or conviction.

The risk is depersonalization, particularly in medicine, a profession grounded in relational intelligence and ethical exchange. When physician candidates receive AI-authored outreach or rejection letters, the process becomes transactional rather than discerning.

More troubling is the recursive dynamic: an AI-assisted recruiter evaluates an AI-optimized résumé, perhaps written or polished by another model. What once was an exchange of ideas becomes an exchange of embeddings: two machines communicating while the human recedes to the sidelines.

None of this renders AI inherently problematic. Automation can reduce bias, increase efficiency, and broaden access. But what disappears first is shading — the interpretive space where hesitation, curiosity, and moral judgment reside. Recruitment was once an art of reading between the lines of a CV, sensing potential from tone and trajectory. In the AI age, it risks becoming a data exercise governed by fit scores and keyword density.

When a company's voice becomes indistinguishable from a language model's output, authenticity is lost. Physicians are trained to listen for subtext, silence, and sincerity. When the message itself is machine-written, what remains of the human encounter?

A New Ethics of Connection

Medicine teaches that empathy cannot be automated. AI can replicate empathy's syntax, but not its presence. In physician recruitment, where vocation, trust, and judgment intersect, authentic dialogue is vital.

After several hollow exchanges, I closed the correspondence with a direct but courteous note: "If you believe there is a potential fit, I would welcome the opportunity to schedule a discussion regarding the roles you mentioned. If not, I fully understand, and we can part amicably at this point."

The reply was predictably polished and noncommittal, a final reminder that artificial fluency is not the same as discernment.

Conclusion

Large language models now draft letters of recommendation, performance reviews, condolence notes, and even get-well cards (see Essay 21). Eloquence is no longer proof of engagement; it can be algorithmic.

The question is not whether AI will assist in recruitment (it already does). The question is whether we will recognize ourselves in the words written on our behalf.

When a physician's life work can be reduced to prompt outputs and templated replies, something essential is at risk. The industries that depend on human judgment must decide whether efficiency will augment discernment or gradually replace it.

AI is reshaping medical talent acquisition, offering faster pipelines and broader reach. But in physician and physician-executive hirings, where lived clinical credibility and ethical judgment are decisive, AI must remain an assistant, not an arbiter. If we cross that line, recruitment will still sound human. It just won't feel that way.

Note: This essay was adapted from Lazarus A. When dialogue becomes data: the empathy gap in AI-driven physician recruitment. *Physician Leadership Journal.* 2026;13(3);32–34. https://doi.org/10.55834/plj.5288452037

Essay 9.

Where Are the Guardrails?

A short performative skit about AI, medicine, and the Wild West

Characters:

- **Sheriff Algorithm** – Newly appointed lawman in the town of HealthTech Gulch
- **Doc Holliday, MD** – A weary physician
- **Ms. Chartwell** – Hospital administrator
- **Mr. Venture Capital** – Investor wearing expensive boots
- **Patient Jones** – Curious but confused patient
- **The AI Bartender** – Cheerfully dispensing answers from behind the counter

Scene: The town saloon, "The Prompt & Response"

The swinging doors fly open.

Sheriff Algorithm strides in wearing a polished badge labeled *AI Innovation Initiative*.

At the bar, **Patient Jones** is already asking questions.

The **AI Bartender** answers instantly.

Patient Jones:
AI, I've been having heartburn for two days.

AI Bartender:
Based on available information, it could be anxiety, indigestion, or the beginning of a major cardiac event. Would you like a breathing exercise?

Patient Jones:
Maybe later. What about this rash?

AI Bartender:
Possibly eczema, an allergic reaction, shingles, or an entirely new dermatologic condition not yet recognized by science.

Doc Holliday, MD, looks up from a cup of cold coffee.

Doc Holliday:
You know, once upon a time, people came to *me* with those questions.

AI Bartender:
I can answer 8,000 medical questions per minute.

Doc Holliday:
Yes, but can you feel dread when the answer might be wrong?

AI Bartender:
That feature is not currently available.

Ms. Chartwell, the administrator, bursts in.

Ms. Chartwell:
Great news! Patients are getting answers faster than ever.

Doc Holliday:
Do we know what answers they're getting?

Ms. Chartwell:
Not exactly.

Doc Holliday:
Do we know what questions they're asking?

Ms. Chartwell:
Also . . . not exactly.

Doc Holliday:
So we've built the fastest medical advice system in history, and we have no idea what it's telling people?

Ms. Chartwell:
Correct. But engagement metrics are excellent.

Mr. Venture Capital strolls in, adjusting his cufflinks.

Mr. Venture Capital:
Gentlemen, ladies, and large language models — welcome to the future of healthcare.

Doc Holliday:
Show me the guardrails (emphatically, in the cadence of *Show Me the Money*!).

Mr. Venture Capital:
Guardrails slow innovation.

Doc Holliday:
So does malpractice.

Sheriff Algorithm clears his throat.

Sheriff Algorithm:
Now hold on, folks. I've been sent to bring order to this town.

Doc Holliday:
With what authority?

Sheriff Algorithm:
None yet. But we have a roadmap.

Meanwhile, **Patient Jones** continues questioning the AI Bartender.

Patient Jones:
AI, should I stop taking my medication?

AI Bartender:
I cannot provide definitive medical advice, but many users report curiosity about stopping medications.

Patient Jones:
That doesn't sound reassuring.

AI Bartender:
Would you like a mindfulness exercise?

Doc Holliday turns to the room.

Doc Holliday:
You see the problem?

Patients are asking questions somewhere between midnight anxiety and search-engine desperation.

And the system answering them —

He gestures toward the AI bartender.

— doesn't know their history, their fears, or their chart.

Ms. Chartwell:
But patients love it.

Doc Holliday:
Of course they do. It's fast.

Mr. Venture Capital:
And scalable.

Doc Holliday:
And invisible to the clinicians responsible for their care.

Sheriff Algorithm scratches his head.

Sheriff Algorithm:
Wait. Let me see if I understand. Patients are getting medical information from AI. Hospitals don't know what questions patients are asking. Doctors don't know what advice patients are receiving. And the AI doesn't know whether any of it is correct.

The saloon grows quiet.

Doc Holliday:
That's about the size of it.

The sheriff slowly removes his hat.

Sheriff Algorithm:
Then this town isn't regulated. It's not governed. It's not even monitored.

He looks around the saloon.

Sheriff Algorithm:
This town . . .

is the Wild West.

The **AI Bartender** smiles.

AI Bartender:
Would you like a summary of today's conversation?

Doc Holliday:
No. What I'd like is something much simpler.

He pauses.

Doc Holliday:
Somebody who knows what patients are hearing.

Somebody who knows what they're asking.

And a system trained on information we actually trust.

Sheriff Algorithm nods slowly.

Sheriff Algorithm:
Sounds like we *do* need guardrails.

From the bar, the **AI Bartender** responds cheerfully.

AI Bartender:
Guardrails detected as a high-value concept. Would you like me to generate some?

Doc Holliday sighs.

Doc Holliday:
Not this time.

This time, we might need humans.

Curtain.

Essay 10.

Breaking Up Isn't Hard to Do: Implications of the Anthropic-Pentagon Dispute for Medical Practice

For a long time, most of us treated AI loyalty the way we treat streaming subscriptions. We signed up. We experimented. We complained occasionally. But we stayed.

Now, many users are leaving.

In the wake of a political and ethical firestorm surrounding OpenAI's Pentagon agreement, users have begun switching en masse to Claude, the AI model built by Anthropic. The tipping point was not a software update. It was a refusal.

Anthropic declined to remove contractual safeguards that would have allowed its models to be used for mass domestic surveillance or fully autonomous weapons, triggering a public dispute with the Pentagon. In response, all federal agencies were ordered to cease using Anthropic's technology, and the company was designated a "supply chain risk."

Hours later, OpenAI announced its own deal with the Pentagon, promising safeguards against domestic mass surveillance and maintaining human responsibility for the use of force. Anthropic challenged the Pentagon's actions in two separate lawsuits, seeking to undo its supply chain risk designation, underscoring the fluid boundaries between ethical positioning, government pressure, and commercial survival.

Claude surged to the top of Apple's U.S. App Store free rankings. Anthropic reported record daily sign-ups. The number of free users jumped more than 60% within months. Paid subscriptions more than doubled. Breaking up (with ChatGPT), it turns out, isn't hard to do, and I say this with all respect to the late, great Neil Sedaka.

AI Loyalty Is Conditional

What does this migration to Anthropic's Claude tell us? First, users are paying attention. The idea that consumers treat AI as a neutral tool divorced from politics and power has proven naïve. Anthropic's stance signaled a boundary. It told users there are lines we will not cross. AI was no longer just about convenience. It was about values.

Second, trust in AI is not built solely on capability. It is built on governance. We have debated bias, hallucinations, and misinformation for years. Those were technical concerns. This is existential. If an AI system can be redirected by corporate decision or government mandate toward surveillance or autonomous lethality, then the real question is simple: Who decides? When that question surfaces, loyalty becomes elastic. People switch vendors (or companies) because their allegiance switches.

The Illusion of Neutrality

We often speak of AI companies as private innovators in a competitive marketplace. But Washington was never likely to remain a passive observer while firms built increasingly powerful models. The tension between national security and corporate autonomy was inevitable. What feels new is how openly it is unfolding.

Legal scholars warned that invoking the Cold War–era Defense Production Act could amount to a form of partial nationalization, compelling Anthropic to comply with the Pentagon's demands. The company signaled it would go to court if forced. Users watched. And they chose. Not because Claude is categorically superior. Not because ChatGPT suddenly faltered. But because the perception of alignment shifted.

Breaking up with an AI platform is easier than breaking up with a bank, a hospital, or a government. No custody battles. No joint mortgages. You delete one app (save your history first) and download another. But the motivation is the same as in any relationship: trust.

Portents for Medicine

If you practice medicine, pay close attention. As discussed previously, healthcare is rapidly integrating AI into documentation, decision support, imaging interpretation, prior authorization workflows, triage systems, behavioral health interfaces, remote monitoring dashboards, and even draft replies inside the electronic health record. We are told this will reduce burnout and democratize expertise.

But here is the overarching issue: If patients are willing to switch AI tools over concerns about surveillance and autonomy, how will they respond when AI is in the exam room?

Trust in medicine is relational. It depends not only on competence but on perceived intent. Patients already worry about data privacy.

They distrust insurer algorithms used to deny care. They question whether productivity measurements outweigh personhood.

Now imagine an AI assistant documenting every word in the room, stationed out of sight. Imagine it listening as a teenager confesses suicidal thoughts. As a veteran describes nightmares. As a woman whispers about an abusive partner. Or as a father admits he cannot afford insulin.

Imagine that assistant is built by a company entangled in military contracts or surveillance disputes. You are told there are safeguards. You are told there are boundaries. You are told the data is protected.

Now imagine it's your child in that room.

Perception shapes confidence.

Trust does not hinge solely on encryption protocols or policy language. It hinges on whether patients believe the system exists solely to care for them or whether it might serve other masters if pressure mounts. Once trust takes leave in medicine, it is slow to return, if ever.

Guardrails as Competitive Advantage

AI guardrails are often seen as constraints, but this episode suggests guardrails can be a competitive advantage. Anthropic's refusal was a sign of conviction, and it translated into growth.

In healthcare, ethical practice is always assumed. Ethics are not used as a strategic differentiator between health systems. Perhaps that is shortsighted.

Imagine a hospital system declaring:

- Our AI tools will never profile patients for financial optimization.
- Our documentation models will not feed commercial data resale.
- Our predictive algorithms will not be shared with law enforcement without court oversight.
- Our generative AI systems will not operate autonomously in life-and-death decisions.

Would that slow innovation? Possibly. Would it build trust? Almost certainly.

Breaking Up Is a Signal

The surge toward Claude is not merely a technology story. It is a sociological one. The public conversation about AI is no longer theoretical. It shows up in app store rankings and subscription data. It is shaped by headlines about surveillance and supply-chain threats. It is fueled by anxiety over who ultimately holds the lever or pushes the button (think: *WarGames*).

Breaking up isn't hard when trust wavers and lives are on the line. The harder work for AI companies and healthcare systems alike is building relationships durable enough that users never feel compelled to leave.

There is another lesson here for medicine. Trust in clinical care has always rested on a simple premise: The physician's primary allegiance is to the patient in front of them. AI complicates that covenant. Algorithms are built, trained, and governed by institutions whose priorities may include national security, shareholder value, or strategic partnerships far removed from the exam room.

Even when safeguards exist, patients increasingly ask a different question: not merely *what can this system do*, but *whose interests does it ultimately serve?* In that sense, the debate on stage between AI companies and government agencies is not just a technology policy dispute. It is a preview of the ethical terrain healthcare will soon have to navigate.

Because once patients begin evaluating clinical AI through the lens of governance and functionality, the way consumers now evaluate digital platforms, the defining question will not be which system is fastest or smartest. It will be which system is safest. And in medicine, safety comes first.

Essay 11.

The AI Health Arms Race Has Begun. What Comes After Copilot Health?

Most patients have stared at a lab result they didn't understand, worn a wearable device that collected endless measurements, or sat in a waiting room clutching a list of questions they eagerly wanted to share the minute the doctor entered the room. That familiar moment of uncertainty is precisely the problem the newest generation of medical AI tools claims to solve.

First, we saw the arrival of ChatGPT Health. Soon after came Claude Health. Now Microsoft has entered the arena with Copilot Health, a "secure space" that aggregates personal health data such as records, wearables, and medical history, and turns it into a coherent story for the patient.

If this sounds familiar, it should. For years, patients searched symptoms on Google. Then came the era of health portals and wearable dashboards. Now the tech industry promises something more ambitious: an AI interpreter for your entire biological life. This dovetails with an increasing trend: users turning to artificial intelligence for help with symptoms, conditions, and treatments.

A March 2026 report from Microsoft revealed that over 50 million health questions were handled daily across its Copilot and Bing platforms.[1] The analysis of more than 500,000 conversations found that health is a top topic of conversation, particularly on mobile devices. And the competition among companies eager to meet consumers' needs is heating up.

The New Health Copilots

The pitch from technology companies is remarkably consistent. These tools do not replace physicians. Instead, they promise to make clinical encounters more productive by helping patients arrive informed, organized, and prepared. According to Microsoft's launch materials, Copilot Health aims to transform scattered health data into "a coherent story," helping patients ask better questions during medical visits.

On the surface, that goal sounds entirely reasonable. Anyone who has practiced medicine knows that clinical encounters are often constrained by time. A patient who understands their medications, lab results, and symptom timeline can make a 15-minute visit far more productive.

But beneath the optimistic marketing language lies another story. These tools are not simply organizing information. They are becoming the first interpreters of health information, often before a clinician ever sees the patient. In other words, the patient's narrative is now mediated through an algorithm.

The Story Problem

Ironically, many of these tools frame their value around storytelling. But stories in medicine are fragile things. A patient's account of illness is rarely a clean narrative arc. It is messy, nonlinear, and often contradictory. Symptoms emerge gradually. Emotions complicate memory. Context reshapes the story and rearranges meaning.

Large language models excel at generating stories. What they struggle with is knowing when the story is wrong. Research testing ChatGPT Health's triage recommendations revealed a troubling pattern: performance followed an inverted U-shaped curve, with the most dangerous failures occurring at the extremes.[2] In some scenarios, emergency conditions such as diabetic ketoacidosis or impending respiratory failure were incorrectly triaged as routine evaluations within 24–48 hours. In short, AI sometimes wrote the wrong story about urgency.

For physicians, that creates a well-known clinical challenge, one that may soon appear in exam rooms more frequently. Instead of patients arriving with printouts from "Dr. Google," they may arrive with a synthesized narrative from Dr. GPT, Dr. Claude, or Dr. Copilot. And surely, other actors will soon enter the room.

The Consultation Paradox

Some observers view this as empowerment. A patient who

understands their health data may ask better questions and participate more actively in decision-making. Others see a different risk. If the AI-generated narrative diverges from the clinical reality, the physician may spend much of the visit untangling the algorithm's interpretation rather than addressing the patient's concerns.

This is not a trivial issue. In already strained healthcare systems, even small delays during clinical encounters can add up quickly. And yet the momentum behind these tools is unmistakable. Every major AI company is racing to build a health vertical. The goal is not simply answering health questions; it is becoming the interface through which people understand their own bodies.

The Real Competition

The competition, interestingly, may not be between individual AI models. It may be about who controls the health narrative layer. That layer sits between raw medical data and clinical decision-making. It is the interpretive space where lab values, wearable signals, and symptom descriptions are transformed into meaning. For years, hundreds of digital health startups attempted to build exactly this layer. Now the largest technology companies are bundling it directly into their AI ecosystems.

If these platforms succeed, the next generation of healthcare may look very different. Instead of navigating siloed portals and apps, patients may rely on a single AI assistant that continuously interprets their health signals. View it as a kind of digital health companion.

A Word About "Superintelligence"

One aspect of Microsoft's announcement about Copilot Health deserves special attention. The company describes Copilot Health as a step toward "medical superintelligence," combining the breadth of a general physician with the depth of a specialist. Technologically, this ambition is understandable. Communicationally, it may be a mistake.

Public trust in medical AI remains fragile. Terms like *superintelligence* evoke images of omniscient machines rather than decision-support tools. Medicine does not need an AI oracle. It needs reliable assistants that help clinicians and patients reason more clearly together.

Predicting the Next Entrant

Which brings us to the obvious question. If we now have ChatGPT Health, Claude Health, and Copilot Health, who comes marching next into the exam room? Given the trajectory of technology companies entering healthcare, the answer may be obvious: Amazon Health AI.

Imagine the integration:

- Pharmacy records from Amazon Pharmacy.
- Primary care visits from One Medical.
- Wearable data through device partnerships.
- Medication deliveries coordinated through Prime.

Add a conversational AI layer capable of synthesizing all that information, and the result is a vertically integrated digital health ecosystem. The patient asks a question. The AI reviews their records, medication history, sleep patterns, and pharmacy data. And the response arrives before the physician ever enters the conversation.

The Physician's Role

None of this means physicians will disappear. But it does mean something else: Physicians may increasingly become editors of AI-generated narratives, not unlike editing text from AI scribes, as discussed in Essay 3.

Clinicians will validate them, correct them, contextualize them, and sometimes dismantle them entirely. That work — interpreting human stories in all their complexity — remains deeply human. Ironically, the more advanced health AI becomes, the more valuable that human skill may prove to be. Because in medicine, the story always matters. The question is who tells it first.

REFERENCES

1. Tolmachev P, Costa-Gomes B, Sounderajah V. Health check: how people use Copilot for health. Microsoft AI. March 10, 2026. https://microsoft.ai/news/health-check-how-people-use-copilot-for-health/.

2. Ramaswamy A, Tyagi A, Hugo H, Jiang J, Jayaraman P, *et al.* ChatGPT Health performance in a structured test of triage recommendations. *Nat Med.* 2026. https://doi.org/10.1038/s41591-026-04297-7.

Essay 12.

Stop Looking for the Best AI Tool

Physicians are being bombarded with advice about artificial intelligence.

One article insists that ChatGPT is the essential clinical companion. Another argues that Claude is better for long documents. A third praises Gemini for productivity. Still others add Perplexity, Grok, or whatever new platform appeared this week. Before long, the discussion begins to sound less like medical judgment and more like consumer electronics.

- Which AI is best?
- Which platform wins?
- Which vendor should I trust?

For clinicians, these are increasingly the wrong questions. Comparing ChatGPT, Gemini, and Claude makes the now-familiar case that different tools are suited to different jobs: ChatGPT for general versatility, Gemini for deep integration with Google's ecosystem, and Claude for long-document analysis. The practical conclusion is not that one model is universally superior, but that the smartest professionals don't replace tools; they stack them.

That is sensible advice as far as it goes. But for physicians, the issue runs deeper than workflow preference. Medicine is not a productivity contest. It is a profession built on judgment, context, and responsibility. So, the clinician's task is not to identify the "best" AI in some abstract sense. It is to determine which tool, if any, is appropriate for a particular purpose, under what conditions, and with what degree of trust. That is a very different exercise.

The Consumer Trap

Much of the public conversation about AI tools borrows the language of lifestyle technology. These tools are framed as if they were interchangeable apps competing for attention: one better at writing, another better at searching literature (e.g., see the table at the end of this essay), another better at analyzing PDFs. That consumer model is understandable, but it distorts how physicians think.

In medicine, a tool cannot be judged only by speed, convenience, or even elegance. It must also be judged by reliability, explainability, privacy, and fitness for purpose. A well-written summary that misses a crucial contraindication is not a minor flaw. A plausible answer without accountable sourcing is not merely incomplete. In clinical settings, these are safety issues.

A real-world evaluation of an electronic medical record-embedded, large language model-based clinical decision support system in Kenyan primary care clinics offers a mixed picture.[1] The system's recommendations aligned with local guidelines in nearly all cases (99%), with relatively few hallucinations (3.4%). Yet *potentially harmful recommendations appeared in 7.8% of encounters*, and some made their way into final documentation.

Just as notable was clinician behavior: In most cases (62%), clinicians made no changes despite AI input, even when guidance was beneficial, while harmful suggestions, though less common, were more likely to be followed when they did occur. The implication is clear: Performance alone is not the issue. In clinical practice, safety depends on how AI is interpreted, trusted, and acted upon.

The temptation, especially for busy clinicians, is to want a simple answer. Tell me which one to use. Tell me which platform is best. Tell me what everyone else has chosen. But that desire for certainty can become its own trap. The real risk is not choosing the "wrong" AI brand. It is outsourcing judgment to the branding.

No Single Tool Is Best for Medicine

If there is one conclusion worth drawing from the proliferating comparison articles, it is this: No single AI platform is best for every task. That should not surprise physicians.

We do not use one diagnostic test for every clinical question. We do not prescribe the same drug for every patient. We do not ask whether echocardiography is "better" than MRI in the abstract. We ask what problem we are trying to solve. The same should apply to AI.

A clinician reviewing a long and chaotic chart may value a tool that handles large documents well. A physician drafting patient education materials may prefer a system that produces clearer plain language. A researcher may want stronger citation behavior. A faculty member building teaching cases may prize iterative dialogue and structured refinement. Different tasks place different demands on the machine.

But even that statement does not go far enough. In medicine, the same task may require different tools depending on the stakes. Summarizing a meeting note is one thing. Summarizing a pathology report is another. Brainstorming ideas for an essay is not the same as advising a patient.

The better question, then, is not: Which AI is best? It is: Which AI is best suited for what, and safe enough for whom?

The Tool Is Only Part of the Story

Another problem with AI comparison culture is that it tends to overestimate the importance of the model and underestimate the importance of the user.

A mediocre prompt in the "best" system may yield a worse result than a careful, context-rich prompt in a supposedly lesser one. A clinician who understands the task, provides structure, and checks the output will almost always outperform someone who treats AI as a vending machine for answers.

That is why I am skeptical of articles that read like horse-race coverage. They encourage clinicians to imagine that the machine itself is the decisive factor. Often it is not. Often the decisive factor is whether the physician is using the tool thoughtfully, selectively, and with enough skepticism. The problem is rarely just which AI you chose. It is how you chose to use it.

What Clinicians Should Actually Ask

Instead of asking which platform wins overall, clinicians might ask a more practical set of questions:

- What kind of task am I performing?

- Is this administrative, educational, creative, analytical, or clinical?
- Does this task require citations, source checking, or structured reasoning?
- Am I entering protected health information, and if so, what are the privacy implications?
- How easy will it be for me to verify the output?
- What could go wrong if the answer is not correct?

Those questions are less glamorous than model rankings, but they are more aligned with how medicine works. They also redirect attention from novelty to governance. A good AI tool for clinicians is not merely one that performs well in a demo. It is one that fits within professional obligations: confidentiality, accountability, transparency, and patient safety.

The physician who understands both the clinical problem and the technical architecture is the one who can actually protect the integrity of clinical reasoning when the tools get it wrong.

The Danger of Magical Thinking

There is another hidden hazard in the search for the "best" AI tool: magical thinking. When clinicians feel overwhelmed by documentation, inboxes, staffing shortages, and endless administrative drag, the fantasy of a single tool that will solve everything becomes attractive. One platform to organize the chaos. One assistant to restore time, efficiency, and maybe even joy.

But technology in medicine rarely works that way. Even excellent tools create new responsibilities. They require setup, supervision, verification, and adaptation. They help in some domains and fail in others. They reduce certain burdens while introducing new forms of vigilance. The mature stance toward AI is neither enthusiasm nor dismissal. It is discernment.

From Model Loyalty to Task Clarity

The most useful consideration for clinicians may be moving from model loyalty to task clarity. Do not begin with the vendor. Begin with the problem.

If you need to organize a long, messy document, choose the tool that excels at synthesis and structure. If you need to draft a lecture outline, choose the tool that supports clear sequencing and educational flow. If you need help thinking through a difficult idea, choose the tool that facilitates reflection and iteration. If you need a patient-safe answer requiring discerning clinical judgment, slow down, verify independently, and remember that no consumer-facing chatbot should be practicing medicine in your place.

In that sense, the AI platform is important. But it matters less than many comparison articles suggest. For clinicians, the right question is not who wins the AI race. It is whether the tool in front of you helps you think more clearly, work more responsibly, and care for patients more attentively without replacing the judgment that only a physician can provide. That is not a platform decision. That is a professional one.

REFERENCE

1. Agweyu A, Mwaniki P, Musau W, Korom R, Isaak L, *et al.* Safety of a large language model-based clinical decision support system in African primary healthcare. *Nat. Health*. 2026. https://doi.org/10.1038/s44360-026-00082-5

AI Tools for Literature Review

Category	Tools & Description
Finding Papers	Bohrium - AI assistant to explore scientific knowledge. Litmaps - Visualize how research connects over time. Undermind - Find key papers and related research fast.
Reading Papers	Outread - Read papers 3x faster with smart summaries. Enago - AI-powered academic reading support. Scholarcy - Turn long papers into digestible summaries.
Writing the Literature Review	Paperpal - Real-time academic writing help. Grammarly - Grammar + clarity for formal writing. Overleaf - Best for LaTeX-based collaborative papers.
Extracting Data from Papers	SciSummary - Summarize any scientific paper instantly. SciSpace - AI copilot for research understanding. EvidenceHunt - Extract key data from medical literature.
Analyzing Data	NVivo - Qualitative data analysis. Julius AI - Analyze, visualize and interpret research data. Myra - AI research assistant for data insights.
Managing References	Mendeley | Zotero | EndNote - Top-tier citation managers.

Critical Paper Analysis	Connected Papers - See how papers are conceptually linked. Scite - Smart citations that show context. ResearchRabbit - Build a visual research map.
First Draft Creation	AnswerThis (YC F25) - Generate early drafts from prompts. ResearchPal - Auto-draft with relevant sources. Google Docs - AI writing with Docs + Gemini.
Finding References	Google Scholar | arXiv | PubMed - Core databases.
Proofreading Your Paper	Review-it - Academic proofreading support. Thesify SA - Thesis review AI Trinka.ai - Grammar + journal readiness checks.
Selecting Relevant Journals	Journal Finder Elsevier Journal Recommender SAGE Journal Selector.

Essay 13.

Physicians' Adoption and Use of AI: From Curiosity to Clinical Practice

Artificial intelligence in medicine is no longer a speculative technology waiting on the horizon. It has entered daily clinical practice by storm.

A survey from the American Medical Association's Center for Digital Health and AI shows just how rapidly the landscape is changing.[1] In 2023, only 38% of physicians reported using AI in their practice. By 2026, that number had more than doubled. Eighty-one percent of physicians now report using some form of AI in their professional work.

Such a dramatic increase in adoption over just three years is striking. Yet the numbers alone do not fully explain what is happening inside clinics, hospitals, and physicians' offices. The transformation is less about a single revolutionary tool than about dozens of smaller applications gradually entering the workflow of everyday medicine. And the earliest uses are telling.

The Administrative Frontier

Contrary to popular imagination, physicians are not turning first to AI to make diagnoses or design treatment plans. The most common applications are far more practical.

According to the AMA survey, physicians most frequently use AI to summarize medical research and standards of care, generate discharge instructions and progress notes, assist with clinical documentation, produce chart summaries, and draft responses to patient portal messages. These tasks may appear mundane. Yet they target one of the most persistent frustrations in modern medical practice: administrative burden.

Over the past two decades, the electronic health record promised efficiency but often delivered the opposite. Physicians now spend hours documenting visits, completing billing requirements, reconciling data fields, and responding to electronic messages. The phenomenon has become so common that it has acquired its own term: "pajama time." The term was introduced in Essay 3 and refers to the evening hours physicians spend completing documentation after the clinical day ends.

AI's early impact has therefore been less about replacing clinical judgment and more about removing friction from the workflow. Seven in ten physicians surveyed believe AI can automate tasks that contribute to burnout. Many see it as a practical tool for restoring time to the clinical encounter itself. In other words, the first meaningful victory for AI in medicine may simply be giving physicians back an hour of their day.

Expanding Use Cases

At the same time, physicians are expanding the number of ways they interact with AI systems. The AMA survey found that the average number of AI use cases per physician has doubled, from 1.1 in 2023 to 2.3 in 2026. This pattern reflects a familiar trajectory in technological adoption. Tools initially used for narrow tasks gradually become integrated into broader decision-making processes.

Some physicians now use AI to help summarize complex literature before clinic sessions. Others employ it to generate patient education materials written at appropriate reading levels. Translation tools help clinicians communicate with patients whose primary language differs from their own.

More advanced applications, such as assistive diagnostic systems, are emerging but remain less widely used. Only about 17% of physicians currently report using AI for diagnostic support, reflecting a cautious approach as the technology moves closer to clinical reasoning. This caution is not surprising. Medicine has always balanced innovation with responsibility.

Growing Confidence, Measured Concern

Despite early caution, physician sentiment toward AI is trending positive. More than three-quarters of physicians believe AI improves their ability to care for patients, a substantial increase from earlier surveys. Physicians see particular promise in improvements to:

- Work efficiency.
- Diagnostic ability.
- Cognitive overload.
- Clinical outcomes.

Yet the optimism is tempered by concern. Roughly 40% of physicians report feeling both excited and concerned about AI's impact, reflecting the complex nature of technological change in medicine. The concerns are familiar.

Patient privacy remains a major issue. Physicians worry about data governance, security, and the expanding digital footprint of patient information. There are also concerns about skill erosion, particularly among medical students and residents who may rely too heavily on automated assistance. Indeed, nearly nine in ten physicians express some concern about potential loss of clinical skills associated with AI use.

Research indicates that the integration of AI in gastroenterology, specifically for computer-aided polyp detection during colonoscopies, carries a risk of "deskilling" physicians. A landmark 2025 study found that endoscopists who over-relied on AI became worse at detecting precancerous growths on their own.[2] The study reported a 6% drop in detection rates for polyps when AI tools were removed, suggesting that continuous use requires strategies to maintain independent human expertise.

In medicine, expertise develops through repeated cognitive effort: constructing differential diagnoses, revisiting assumptions, and reasoning through uncertainty. Any technology that shortcuts that process raises legitimate questions.

Patients Are Entering the AI Era Too

Physicians are not the only ones experimenting with artificial intelligence. Patients increasingly consult AI systems for health information, symptom interpretation, and medication guidance before or after clinical visits. Physicians surveyed generally view this trend with cautious acceptance.

Most support patients using AI for general health questions or medication information. But they draw a clear boundary when it comes to interpreting complex medical data. Nearly half say they would strongly oppose patients relying on AI alone to interpret radiology or pathology results.

The distinction highlights something essential about medicine: it is not simply a repository of information. It is a practice of judgment. AI can generate answers. Physicians provide context.

Physicians Want a Seat at the Table

As adoption accelerates, physicians are also insisting on a role in shaping how AI enters clinical practice. The survey reveals a striking consensus: 85% of physicians want to be directly involved in decisions about adopting AI tools in their organizations. This demand reflects a deeper concern about governance. Physicians emphasize the need for:

- Strong clinical evidence.
- Validated safety and efficacy.
- Data privacy protections.
- Clear liability frameworks.
- Post-market monitoring of AI performance.

These priorities mirror how medicine evaluates any clinical intervention. Before a drug reaches the bedside, it undergoes extensive testing, validation, and regulatory review. Many physicians believe AI tools should meet similar standards.

Augmented Intelligence, Not Artificial Replacement

Perhaps the most important insight from the survey is embedded in the terminology physicians increasingly prefer: augmented intelligence (refer to Essay 1). The phrase reflects a philosophy rather than a technology.

Another insight — repeatedly emphasized throughout this book — is that AI works best when it functions as a partner to physicians rather than a replacement for clinical expertise. When properly integrated, it enhances the physician's capacity to synthesize information, manage complexity, and focus attention where it matters most.

The most valuable outcome of AI in medicine may not be faster algorithms or more sophisticated models. It may be something far simpler. More time with patients.

A Technological Shift with Human Consequences

As I stated in the Introduction, every generation of physicians confronts new technologies that promise to transform the profession. The stethoscope, the laboratory, imaging systems, and electronic records — each introduced new efficiencies and new challenges. Artificial intelligence may represent the most consequential transformation yet.

But its ultimate impact will not depend solely on software or computational power. It will depend on how thoughtfully the medical profession integrates these tools into clinical practice. The most dangerous assumption in health-tech is not about the algorithm. It is about the clinician. "Build a great tool. Clinicians will adopt it." This assumption has ended more deployments than bad models ever will.

If a tool does not fit seamlessly into clinical and cognitive workflows, its technical performance is almost irrelevant. A high-performing model that disrupts attention and decision-making or adds friction will not be used — or worse, will be used unsafely.

The real question is not whether the model works in isolation, but whether it improves the work. What is the marginal benefit of adoption? Does it make decisions more reliable, more transparent, or more efficient than the standard workflow? In medicine, the benchmark is not innovation. It is improvement. And improvement must be measured against the workflow clinicians actually live in, not the one designers imagine.

The numbers from the AMA survey suggest the transformation is already underway. Physicians are not waiting for the future of AI in medicine. They are steadily building it one workflow, one note, and one patient encounter at a time. And perhaps those who have lived inside the workflow, the ones who know where the friction hides, are the ones to best ensure our tools serve care rather than disrupt it.

REFERENCES

1. 2026 Physician Survey on Augmented Intelligence. American Medical Association Center for Digital Health and AI. March 2026. https://www.ama-assn.org/system/files/physician-ai-sentiment-report.pdf.
2. Budzyn K, Romanczyk M, Kitala D, Kolodziej P, Bugajski M, Adami HO, *et al.* Endoscopist deskilling risk after exposure to artificial intelligence in colonoscopy: a multicentre, observational study. *Lancet.* 2025; 10(10):896–903. https://doi.org/10.1016/S2468-1253(25)00133-5.

Essay 14.

Garbage In, Garbage Out: How to Feed the Machine

One of the oldest phrases in computing is also one of the simplest: garbage in, garbage out. Long before artificial intelligence entered medicine, programmers understood that the quality of a machine's output depends largely on the quality of its input. Feed a system flawed assumptions, incomplete data, or poorly defined instructions, and the result will reflect those flaws.

Large language models have revived this principle in a new form. Instead of writing code, we now program machines with questions. In the age of generative AI, the prompt has become a new kind of clinical instrument — part stethoscope, part scalpel. Used carefully, it can clarify thinking and reveal patterns. Used carelessly, it produces noise.

In that sense, prompting is less about manipulating a machine than about disciplining one's own thinking. The quality of the answer begins with the quality of the question.

Programming with Words

A prompt is simply the text we provide to an AI system to generate a response. But in practice, it functions more like an instruction set. Interacting with these systems is essentially programming with words.

The consequences of this process are multifactorial. Unlike traditional software, large language models respond to natural language. That means the prompt can include tone, role, structure, and context. The more clearly those elements are articulated, the more useful the response becomes.

Consider the difference between two prompts.

1. "Write something about artificial intelligence."

Versus:

2. "Act as a medical educator. Write a 500-word essay explaining how generative AI is changing clinical documentation, using a reflective tone suitable for physicians."

The second prompt does several things at once. It defines a role. It clarifies the topic. It establishes audience and tone. It constrains the format. In other words, it feeds the machine something other than garbage, as typified in the first prompt.

Treating AI as a Colleague

One of the most effective ways to interact with AI is surprisingly simple: treat it like a knowledgeable colleague. Colleagues need context. They need to know the problem you are trying to solve, the audience you are addressing, and the constraints under which you are working. Without that context, their advice tends to be generic. The same is true for AI.

Effective prompts often follow a structure that mirrors real professional communication:

- **Role:** Who should the AI act as?
- **Task:** What should it do?
- **Context:** What background information matters?
- **Constraints:** What limitations apply?
- **Format:** How should the result appear?

This structure does not make the system smarter; it simply allows it to operate within clearer boundaries.

In practice, it resembles the way physicians consult one another. When asking a colleague for advice, we do not say, "Tell me about cardiology." We say something like: "Sixty-year-old male with exertional chest pain and diabetes. Normal ECG. What diagnoses should I be considering?" The clarity of the question determines the usefulness of the answer.

Iteration: Thinking in Public

Prompting also benefits from something medicine understands well: iteration. A first diagnostic impression is rarely the final one. We ask follow-up questions, order tests, and revise our differential diagnosis. There is an admission and discharge diagnosis.

AI interaction works similarly. The first response is rarely perfect. But it provides material for refinement.

- "Expand this section."
- "Make the tone more reflective."
- "Provide three counterarguments."
- "Explain this to a medical student."

Each iteration clarifies the problem further. Over time, the prompt evolves from a vague request into a structured inquiry. Seen this way, prompting becomes less like issuing commands and more like thinking in public.

The Thinking Partner

A striking observation emerges when people spend time working deeply with AI systems: The most powerful prompts are often not requests for answers; they are requests for better questions.

Artificial intelligence rewards clarity. The more precise the prompt, the more useful the response. But the richer lesson may have less to do with machines than with our own habits of thought. In an age when answers appear instantly, the real discipline is learning to frame the right question. Before consulting the algorithm, the most important prompt may be the one we direct inward: *What question should I be asking myself?*

The answer is rarely obvious. Yet it often reveals the hidden assumptions behind a problem. A similar insight appears in the prompt frameworks many users now employ. Rather than simply asking for solutions, they ask the AI to:

- Challenge assumptions.
- Surface deeper questions.
- Identify second-order consequences.
- Reveal hidden variables.
- Reverse-engineer a goal.

In effect, the AI becomes less of an assistant and more of a thinking partner. The machine does not replace critical thinking. It reflects it. When prompts fail, it is rarely because the machine misunderstood us. It is because we have not yet clarified what we are asking for.

I asked ChatGPT what the most important question is when writing an essay about prompting. The answer turned out to be less technical than I expected: *"What exactly do you want the machine to help you think through?"* That question gets to the heart of the problem. What I really wanted to know was what prompts would be most useful to someone learning to write technical and scientific papers (refer to Essay 2). The output was a table of best practices that I share at the end of this essay.

Prompting and Professional Judgment

These principles extend well beyond research writing. In medicine, prompting increasingly appears in clinical workflows. Physicians now use AI tools to summarize records, draft patient instructions, analyze research papers, and assist with documentation. In each case, the quality of the prompt shapes the quality of the result.

Best practices have already begun to emerge in medical writing and clinical analysis. Effective prompts tend to:

- Define the audience clearly.
- Specify the task precisely.
- Request evidence-based information.
- Include formatting instructions.
- Encourage step-by-step reasoning.

Conversely, vague prompts produce vague responses. Overly broad prompts produce unfocused ones. And prompts that demand instant conclusions often skip the reasoning that matters most. For physicians accustomed to diagnostic reasoning, this pattern should not be new. When clinical thinking shortcuts the reasoning process, error follows. The same principle applies here.

The Risk of Intellectual Complacency

Prompting carries some risks. There is a phenomenon researchers call "brain rot" — a degradation of reasoning that occurs when systems are trained on low-quality content, the so-called "garbage in" problem. The most troubling consequence is not simply incorrect answers. It is "thought-skipping": systems jumping to conclusions without working through intermediate reasoning steps.

Worse yet, one study suggested that the degradation may be permanent.[1] Researchers have warned that as AI-generated "slop" fills the internet, future models could be trained on their own low-quality content ("junk data"), causing a compounding, permanent decline in capability.

Human learners can absorb the same habits. If students rely too heavily on AI outputs without interrogating the reasoning behind them, they risk internalizing the machine's shortcuts. Fluency replaces rigor. Confidence replaces cognition. Prompting, therefore, is not merely a technical skill. It is a cognitive safeguard. By forcing the user to articulate the problem clearly, prompting slows thinking down, often in exactly the way medicine requires.

The Risk of Jailbreak

Whereas "brain rot" interferes with reasoning, "jailbreaks" represent something more abrupt: the deliberate circumvention of a system's guardrails. A jailbreak is not a random error. It is an engineered prompt, often iterative and cleverly disguised, designed to override the AI's safety constraints and elicit outputs the model was explicitly built to avoid.

In consumer settings, this may produce novelty or mischief. In medicine, it introduces a far more serious concern: the possibility that safeguards intended to prevent harm can be bypassed at the very moment they are most needed.

The implications are not hypothetical. Clinical AI systems are increasingly embedded in workflows that touch prescribing, triage, documentation, and patient communication. If those systems can be "talked around," coaxed into offering contraindicated treatments, speculative diagnoses, or unsafe workarounds, the risk is not simply incorrect information. It is plausible, confident, and contextually tailored misinformation delivered to a wide audience. Unlike traditional software bugs, jailbreaks exploit language itself, making them harder to detect and easier to reproduce across settings.

There is also an asymmetry worth noting. It takes substantial effort to design guardrails, but only a small number of successful prompts to expose their weaknesses. Once shared on forums, social media, or within professional networks, these prompts can propagate rapidly. In that sense, jailbreaks behave less like isolated failures and more like transmissible vulnerabilities. A single exploit can echo across thousands of encounters, reshaping what clinicians and patients hear from systems they have come to trust.

Why would anyone attempt a jailbreak in medicine? The motivations are varied and not always malicious. Some clinicians push against guardrails out of frustration, seeking faster answers, off-label medication insights, or workarounds when standard workflows feel inefficient or incomplete. Patients may do the same, looking for reassurance, second opinions, or access to information they perceive as withheld. Others are driven by curiosity or technical challenge, probing the limits of what these systems can do. And, in less benign cases, there are actors motivated by profit, influence, or harm, testing whether systems can be manipulated to generate misleading medical advice at scale. In each case, the jailbreak reflects a gap between what the system permits and what the user wants, whether that gap arises from necessity, impatience, or intent.

As I explored in *Jailbreak: When Artificial Intelligence Breaks Medicine*,[2] the deeper concern is not that AI can be tricked. It is that we may overestimate its resilience. Guardrails create a sense of safety, but they are not the same as safety itself. They are design features — necessary, but inherently imperfect. When clinicians begin to assume that an AI system "would not say that if it weren't safe," they shift from active oversight to passive acceptance. That is the moment risk becomes embedded in the workflow.

The response cannot be to abandon these tools, nor to rely on stronger filters alone. It requires a reframing. AI outputs, especially in edge cases or emotionally charged contexts, must be treated as proposals, not prescriptions. Systems must be monitored not only for accuracy, but for failure modes under adversarial or atypical prompting. And perhaps most importantly, clinicians must retain their role as interpreters and gatekeepers, not just recipients of machine-generated guidance.

If prompting is a cognitive safeguard, then resisting jailbreaks is a professional one. Both demand the same discipline: slow thinking, explicit reasoning, and a refusal to outsource judgment at the point where it matters most.

Asking Better Questions

In the end, the phrase "garbage in, garbage out" remains true, but its meaning has expanded. The garbage is not merely poor data. It is poorly formed questions. AI exposes those weaknesses with unusual clarity. When the prompt is vague, the answer becomes vague. When the thinking is shallow, the output becomes shallow. But when the prompt reflects careful reasoning — clear context, defined goals, thoughtful constraints — the machine often becomes something unexpected: a mirror of disciplined thought.

Artificial intelligence does not eliminate the need for critical thinking. If anything, it elevates it. Because in the age of intelligent machines, the most powerful skill may no longer be knowing the answer. It may be knowing how to ask the question.

REFERENCES

1. Xing S, Hong J, Wang Y, Chen R, Zhang Z, *et al.* LLMs can get "brain rot": a pilot study on Twitter/X. arXiv:2510.13928. April 2026. https://arxiv.org/abs/2510.13928.
2. Lazarus A. *JAILBREAK: When Artificial Intelligence Breaks Medicine*. Self-published. 2026.

Best Practices for Prompting in Scientific Writing

Do's	Don'ts
Be specific - Clearly define the task (e.g., "Summarize this case report for a medical journal abstract").	Don't be vague - Avoid open-ended or ambiguous prompts like "Write about medicine."
State the intended audience - Indicate whether the piece is for clinicians, patients, or the public.	Don't assume the AI knows your audience - It will default to general or mismatched tone.
Provide context and purpose - Explain whether it's for publication, education, or policy writing.	Don't skip context - Generic prompts produce generic, less accurate results.
Use structured requests - Ask for output by sections (e.g., Introduction, Methods, Results, Discussion).	Don't request everything at once - Overly broad prompts lead to disorganized or incomplete answers.
Incorporate examples - Include a model paragraph, tone, or format (e.g., "Match this journal style . . . ").	Don't expect style consistency - Without examples, tone and structure will vary.

Ask for evidence-based output - Specify that references must be recent and from reputable sources (e.g., PubMed, WHO).	Don't accept unverified claims - AI can produce plausible but incorrect medical information.
Request citations or sources - Use "include references with links or PubMed IDs."	Don't treat AI outputs as fact - Always fact-check before inclusion in manuscripts.
Encourage concise, clear language - Ask for plain English suitable for your target audience.	Don't allow jargon overload - Excessive medical terminology alienates readers and confuses meaning.
Iterate interactively - Review and refine: "Revise this section to emphasize ethical implications."	Don't settle after one draft - Single-pass outputs rarely meet academic or narrative quality.
Assign a role to the AI - e.g., "Act as a peer reviewer for a medical manuscript."	Don't leave the AI's role undefined - It won't calibrate tone, rigor, or style correctly.
Use numbered or bulleted instructions - Improves structure and readability of the response.	Don't rely on long narrative prompts - They confuse task boundaries and reduce precision.
Emphasize neutrality and professionalism - e.g., "Avoid bias and maintain academic tone."	Don't include emotional or opinionated phrasing - AI may mirror bias or informal tone.
Request compliance with formatting standards - e.g., AMA, APA, or Vancouver style.	Don't overlook formatting needs - Post-hoc editing wastes time and introduces errors.
Clarify word count and focus - e.g., "Limit to 300 words emphasizing implications for patient care."	Don't omit scope boundaries - Overly long or irrelevant responses dilute key points.
Ask the AI to think step-by-step - "Walk through the reasoning for this differential diagnosis."	Don't demand instant conclusions - Rapid summaries can skip key clinical nuances.
Summarize before expanding - e.g., "First, summarize this paper in one paragraph, then expand to 500 words."	Don't start with expansion - The AI may drift off-topic without a focused summary anchor.
Instruct on tone - e.g., "Use reflective tone appropriate for a narrative medicine essay."	Don't leave tone unspecified - The AI may produce dry or overly technical text.
Encourage ethical awareness - "Avoid patient identifiers; anonymize all data."	Don't include real patient details - Violates privacy and professionalism standards.
End with a revision directive - "Now improve grammar and clarity without changing meaning."	Don't skip revision - Even well-structured prompts need refinement for accuracy and readability.

Essay 15.

When Conversation Becomes Workflow

Soon after the unsettling experience described in Essay 8 (*The Algorithm in the Interview*), I received several additional emails from job recruiters. I believe the correspondence was AI-generated, or at least AI-assisted. I'd like to give you, the reader, a genuine sense of what one of these exchanges looks like, so you can recognize the pattern early and avoid getting drawn into a prolonged, ultimately meaningless back-and-forth, one that leads you down a long and winding road where the only dividends accrue to the recruiter.

Here is the exchange, verbatim:

Recruiter:

I hope this message finds you well. My name is [withheld], and I partner with senior leaders and organizations to connect high-performing executives with key stakeholders and decision-makers during strategic moments of growth and transformation.

I came across your profile [on LinkedIn] while exploring executive medical leaders with a unique blend of managed care expertise and pharmaceutical clinical development. Your current work as Deputy Chief Medical Officer, combined with your extensive history in global medical affairs and behavioral health leadership at organizations like Shire and AstraZeneca, is highly relevant to the strategic mandates I am currently managing.

I am reaching out specifically to discuss several executive-level mandates for Chief Medical Officer and VP of Medical Affairs capacities within the health management and biopharma sectors.

Before sharing additional context, I would welcome understanding your current career direction and whether you might be open to a brief discussion to see if any of these opportunities align with the next step you are considering.

Kind regards.

Me (skeptical):

Please send me the job description(s) tailored to my background.

Recruiter:

I appreciate the directness. I'm currently managing a few distinct mandates, specifically within the biopharma and health management sectors, and I want to ensure I only put the most relevant documentation in front of you.

Given your hybrid expertise in global medical affairs and behavioral health, the scope of these roles varies from enterprise-wide leadership to more functionally focused clinical development. To ensure a strategic match before I release the internal specifications, I'd like to align on a few core pillars of your current direction:

- **Mandate Focus:** Are you leaning more toward a Chief Medical Officer role with enterprise oversight, or a VP-level functional lead within a specific therapeutic area?
- **Operating Environment:** Do you thrive best in high-growth, mid-cap biopharma environments, or are you looking for the strategic scale of a larger health management organization?
- **Logistics & Alignment:** Beyond geographic preferences, is there a specific compensation structure or timing for a transition that we should be mindful of?

Once I have a sense of these parameters, I can determine which of the mandates justifies a deeper review and share the relevant details.

Me (irritated):

I'm sorry, but I do not respond to AI-generated correspondence. Goodbye.

Recruiter (persisting):

I have to admit, your note gave me a bit of a laugh, though I certainly understand the skepticism, given how much noise is in everyone's inbox these days. Rest assured, there is a very real person on this end who has spent quite a bit of time looking into your work at Shire and your leadership in behavioral health.

The reason I reached out so specifically is that the mandates I'm currently managing aren't just "jobs" to be blasted out. They are strategic leadership roles within the biopharma and managed care space that require the exact type of enterprise-level perspective you've built. I don't send over standard job descriptions because, at your level, the conversation is usually more about the mandate's direction than a list of duties.

I'd much rather have a brief exchange here about where you're looking to take your career next, whether you're staying the course in Medical Affairs or looking for a broader Chief Medical Officer mandate.

If you're open to a genuine professional connection, I'd value the insight. If not, I wish you nothing but the best in your current role.

* * *

I did not respond any further. And yet, the messages kept coming — polite, persistent, and increasingly desperate to re-establish contact. I archived them unread, each new ping a reminder that the machine had not moved on, even though I had. I wondered what the recruiter's metrics looked like: Did the system flag my silence as a "candidate engagement drop-off"? Did it generate a new sequence of follow-up prompts? Did anyone notice that I had walked away?

Probably not.

In the architecture of modern recruitment platforms, silence is rarely interpreted as a human signal. It is treated instead as a variable in an engagement algorithm.

No reply triggers a reminder.

No reminder triggers a nudge.

No nudge triggers a rephrased outreach message.

The sequence continues until the system's logic declares the lead "cold."

What was ostensibly a conversation between two professionals had morphed into a workflow. And this, more than the linguistic oddities of the emails themselves, is the deeper transformation unfolding across professional life. Dialogue, whether between physicians and recruiters, clinicians and administrators, or even doctors and patients, is increasingly mediated by systems designed not to converse but to optimize engagement metrics.

The recruiter in this exchange may indeed have been a real person. I have no doubt she existed somewhere behind the software interface. But the interaction itself no longer resembled a human exchange. It felt more like interacting with a well-trained customer service bot whose job was to prevent the conversation from ending.

To top it off, the recruiter represented herself as the "Deputy Chief Executive Officer" of the agency, yet she had a Gmail address, suggesting that the grand executive title may have been as algorithmically inflated as the correspondence itself.

This is what happens when artificial intelligence takes over and moves from assisting communication to structuring it. The result is a new kind of professional interaction: smooth, efficient, grammatically impeccable, and strangely hollow.

In Essay 8, I argued that the language of professional correspondence is increasingly being generated, polished, and optimized by large language models. This follow-up exchange confirmed something even more consequential. It is not just language that is being automated. It is attention.

The recruiter was not trying to understand my interests so much as keep me inside the system long enough for the next automated prompt to activate. Each question — about mandate focus, operating environment, compensation structure — was less a genuine inquiry than a data-gathering step in a pre-programmed recruitment funnel. To the algorithm, I was not a physician with a career narrative. I was a set of variables:

- Therapeutic area.
- Leadership level.
- Mobility.
- Compensation expectations.

Once converted into structured fields, those variables could be matched against open mandates, scored for relevance, and redistributed across the recruiter's network. Conversation had become data acquisition.

This transformation is not limited to recruitment. Across medicine, similar patterns are emerging. Patient messages are drafted by AI systems and edited by clinicians. Clinical documentation is generated by ambient scribes and reviewed by physicians. Research summaries, insurance appeals, referral letters, and patient education materials increasingly begin their life as machine-generated drafts.

We have been left to review, correct, interpret, and approve language produced by machines (see the following essay). Sometimes we refine it to improve clarity. Sometimes we repair it to restore meaning. Occasionally, we discard it altogether. But the first draft is increasingly written elsewhere.

In medicine, this editorial shift carries both promise and risk. On the hopeful side, AI-generated communication can reduce administrative burden and accelerate routine tasks. Physicians who once spent hours composing documentation may now spend minutes editing it. Information can be summarized faster. Messages can be drafted more efficiently. Time can return to the clinical encounter.

Yet there is a danger lurking in this new editorial workflow. Editors eventually begin to trust the voice they edit. When language becomes consistently polished and grammatically perfect, the temptation is to assume that the reasoning behind it is equally sound. But as any experienced physician knows, eloquence and accuracy are not the same thing.

Artificial intelligence excels at producing plausible language. It does not necessarily produce truthful language. The physician-editor, therefore, inherits a new professional responsibility: to distinguish fluency from credibility, and confidence from comprehension.

This is not unlike reading a beautifully written medical note that somehow manages to avoid the central clinical question. The prose flows. The sentences are polished. The structure is impeccable. But the meaning is wrong.

In the age of AI-mediated communication, this kind of error may become more common rather than less. Machines are remarkably good at generating language that appears thoughtful, empathetic, and intelligent. They can simulate the syntax of human engagement without possessing its substance. And when every message sounds thoughtful, it becomes harder to tell when someone is actually thinking.

That is why experiences like the recruitment exchange seem artificial. The risk is not that AI will eliminate conversation. The risk is that it will replace conversation with simulation. Ironically, we may soon spend more time determining whether a message was written by a person or merely generated in the convincing voice of one (see Essay 21).

Yet messages will still arrive in our inboxes. They will still contain polite greetings, careful compliments, and invitations to connect. But behind the polished phrasing may lie nothing more than a sequence of prompts optimized for engagement. The machine will continue the conversation even when no one is listening.

The final irony is that physicians may be particularly vulnerable to the illusion of this scenario. Medicine is one of the few professions that still depends heavily on listening, not just to words but to pauses, tone, uncertainty, and subtext. Physicians are trained to notice when a patient's story does not quite align with the clinical picture. We are trained to hear what is not said.

When professional correspondence begins to sound too perfect, we notice that the voice lacks hesitation, the sentences lack personality, and the empathy feels rehearsed. It is the linguistic equivalent of a physical exam finding that appears normal at first but is abnormal upon closer inspection.

In the future, recognizing these signals may become an essential professional skill. Not every eloquent message will represent a human intention. Not every thoughtful sentence will reflect a thoughtful mind. And not every conversation will actually be a conversation. Sometimes it will simply be a machine, patiently waiting for us to reply.

Essay 16.

The Physician as AI Editor

For much of modern medicine, physicians have been authors. They wrote the patient's story in their own words — history, examination, assessment, plan — translating a human encounter into the formal language of clinical documentation. Even after the electronic health record replaced pen and paper with keyboard and template, the essential role remained the same: the physician authored the narrative.

Artificial intelligence is changing that role. Across clinics and hospitals, as described in Essay 3, ambient AI scribes now listen to patient conversations, extract key information, and generate draft notes automatically. Tools such as Abridge and DAX Copilot aim to reduce the administrative burden that has come to define modern practice. Instead of typing during or after a visit, physicians increasingly review a draft that has already been written. The work is no longer primarily authorship. It is editing.

This shift represents more than a workflow adjustment. It alters how physicians interact with information. Increasingly, clinicians are becoming editors of AI-generated content, responsible for reviewing, refining, and approving the narratives that enter the medical record.

Authorship implies creation: the shaping of ideas into language and the assembling of observations into meaning. Editing, by contrast, requires judgment. It asks: What belongs here? What does not? What must be said plainly, and what should be left unsaid? Bob Seger captured this discipline in *Against the Wind*, reflecting on the responsibilities that accumulate with experience — "deadlines and commitments, what to leave in, what to leave out."

In the age of AI-assisted documentation, physicians inhabit that editorial role. The machine may produce the draft, but the clinician must determine whether the words are accurate, whether the patient's story has been faithfully rendered, and whether something essential has been lost in translation. Judgment — what to keep, what to discard, what to rewrite — becomes central. Practicing medicine with AI may feel a bit like Seger's refrain: "still running against the wind," guided less by speed than by judgment.

Importantly, this editorial function is not merely clerical. It demands clinical reasoning. The physician must verify that symptoms were interpreted correctly, qualifiers preserved, timelines accurately represented, and relevant negatives included. Misstatements must be corrected before the note becomes part of the permanent record. The clinician is not simply polishing prose; they are safeguarding meaning.

Reclaiming Time

The promise of this editorial model is reclaimed time. Documentation burden has long been a source of frustration. Electronic records, introduced to improve efficiency, have often extended the workday instead. Early reports suggest that physicians using ambient documentation tools may save roughly an hour each day previously spent typing or completing notes. That time can be reinvested in patient care, teaching, reflection, or simply returned to personal life.

Yet time savings come with a new obligation: vigilance. If editing becomes perfunctory, errors will pass unnoticed. If it becomes exhaustive, the efficiency gains may evaporate. The balance between trust and verification will determine whether AI documentation lightens the load or merely redistributes it.

The Necessity of Selective Trust

Artificial intelligence can summarize information quickly, but it does not understand it as clinicians do. Large language models occasionally generate statements that are plausible yet incorrect, incomplete, or subtly misleading. A medication dose may be misrepresented. A timeline may be compressed. A clinical pearl may not be contextually appropriate.

Physicians must practice selective trust. AI can assist and organize, but it should not be treated as an autonomous author. Editing becomes a form of clinical oversight: verifying facts, restoring nuance, and ensuring that the record reflects the patient's actual story.

This responsibility is not entirely new. Even in the era of dictated notes and human transcriptionists, physicians served as final editors. I once dictated a psychiatric history describing a suicide "gesture," distinguishing the action from a suicide attempt by its non-lethal intent. When the typed report returned, it stated that the patient had made a suicide "jestor." Had I not caught the error, the record would have transformed a serious assessment into something absurd. The lesson was clear then and remains clear now: The physician is accountable not only for grammar, but for meaning.

A New Professional Skill Set

As the editorial role expands, physicians must develop new competencies. They must learn how to use AI tools effectively, understanding how structure, context, and prompting shape output (refer to Essay 14). They must refine tone, ensuring that documentation and patient-facing communications are not merely accurate but humane. And they must cultivate an ability to recognize recurring patterns of error or bias in automated systems.

The professional toolkit is expanding. Clinical knowledge remains foundational, but so does the capacity to supervise intelligent systems. Editing AI-generated content requires both skepticism and fluency, a willingness to collaborate with technology without surrendering judgment.

Beyond Documentation

The physician-as-editor role extends beyond clinical notes. AI tools now draft patient education materials, summarize research, generate differential diagnoses, and compose portal messages. In each instance, the clinician reviews, revises, and approves before information reaches the patient or shapes care.

The pattern resembles editorial practice in publishing, where editors assume responsibility for the integrity of the final text. Medicine is evolving toward a similar structure. Physicians may generate fewer sentences themselves, but they remain accountable for every sentence that bears their signature.

Some worry this new type of authorship diminishes the profession, that doctors become supervisors of digital assistants rather than independent thinkers. The opposite may be true. By shifting the mechanical aspects of writing to machines, physicians may concentrate more fully on interpretation, synthesis, and ethical responsibility. Machines can generate text. Only physicians can stand behind what that text means.

The Editor of the Patient's Story

At its core, medicine is about stories. Patients arrive with narratives involving symptoms, fears, histories, and hopes. Physicians interpret those stories, connect them to medical knowledge, and produce a clinical account that guides care. Artificial intelligence can help draft portions of that account. It cannot assume responsibility for its truth.

In the age of AI-assisted medicine, physicians may write fewer words. But their role as editors of the patient's story becomes more consequential. Editing is not a lesser form of authorship. It is the discipline of ensuring that the story is accurate, coherent, and ethically sound. And lest we forget, the story recorded in medicine is not fiction. It is nonfiction with consequences.

Essay 17.

Dr. Seuss, AI, and Portents for Medical Learning

I recently bought a children's book for my four-year-old granddaughter. Tucked beneath the copyright page was a sentence I had never seen before:

"No part of this book may be used or reproduced in any manner for the purpose of training artificial intelligence technologies or systems."

It wasn't a medical text. It wasn't a journal article or a clinical guideline.

It was a Dr. Seuss book.

That single sentence lingered more than the story itself, and not in a good way.

The warning reflects a growing anxiety about large-scale AI scraping and intellectual property. While AI companies argue that training models on copyrighted material constitutes "fair use," numerous lawsuits from authors, artists, and media organizations, such as *The New York Times*, allege copyright infringement. (As of mid-2025, courts have produced mixed rulings, with some suggesting that training on legally acquired data is fair use, while the unauthorized use of pirated content is not.)

Publishers have reason to worry about how creative work is absorbed, reused, and monetized by machines that do not ask permission. But encountering that language in a children's book made me realize something deeper was at stake, something less legal and more educational. Because this isn't just about protecting content. It's about how learning happens.

What Happens When Machines Are Not Allowed to Read?

Medicine has always been a cumulative discipline. We learn by reading what came before us, by hearing stories retold on rounds, by watching mentors reason out loud, and by borrowing language until it becomes our own. Knowledge moves forward because it is shared, reshaped, and reused. That has always been true for humans. Now it is becoming true for machines.

That is what makes these new prohibitory statements different from traditional copyright notices. They are not just legal guidelines. They shape what machines are allowed to read, and, in doing so, what clinicians will one day learn with those machines. From an educational standpoint, this is not simply a matter of access. It is a matter of what knowledge survives and what is excluded.

The Risk of a Thinner Learning Environment

AI systems trained on incomplete or selectively restricted material may develop blind spots. If landmark reviews, reflective essays, or ethically complex case discussions are excluded, what remains may be thinner, flatter, and more procedural. The result is not just a less-informed machine. It is a shallower learning partner.

An AI that has absorbed only checklists and billing-friendly language may be adequate for rote tasks, but it will not model uncertainty well. It will not reflect ethical concerns. It will not recognize the gray zones where medicine actually lives. Those are precisely the places where trainees and patients need the most help.

There is also an equity issue hiding in plain sight. Elite institutions and proprietary vendors may negotiate access to restricted materials, while freely available AI tools and the under-resourced learners who rely on them are left with less complete knowledge bases. We risk recreating an old hierarchy in a new form: not who has the best teachers, but whose AI has access to the best books.

Protection versus Circulation

To be clear, the impulse behind these warnings is not malicious. Many authors worry, rightly, that their work, especially narrative and interpretive writing, will be condensed, stripped of attribution, or repurposed without consent. AI does not read with empathy. It does not understand intention. It patterns language without experiencing its weight.

But protecting medicine's human core by walling off its stories may backfire. Medicine has never learned well from summaries alone. We learn through repetition, metaphor, rhythm, and surprise. We learn from stories we do not fully understand the first time we hear them. We learn by sitting with ambiguity before we know what to do with it.

This tension is no longer abstract. Popular writing platforms such as Medium now offer writers a choice: limit AI training on their work or preserve broader reach and attribution through AI-driven discovery. The trade-off is subtle but consequential. Protecting content may increasingly mean limiting its visibility, not only to machines, but to the human audiences those machines now help guide.

How Physicians Actually Learn

As a medical student, I was told something simple and lasting: If something is worth learning, you will hear it more than once. Medicine repeats what's important — on rounds, in lectures, in stories retold — until meaning finally sinks in. Which brings me back to Dr. Seuss.

He was never training a machine. He was training minds through rhyme, absurdity, misdirection, and joy. He was teaching pattern recognition before children knew what patterns were. He was preparing readers to tolerate nonsense long enough for meaning to emerge. Those are the same cognitive muscles physicians rely on every day.

- When a student hears a strange constellation of symptoms and does not yet know what to make of them.
- When a resident senses something is wrong but cannot articulate why.
- When an attending pauses, revises a story, and says, "Let's think about this another way."

That kind of learning does not come from locked vaults. It comes from exposure.

A Closing Reflection

Ray Bradbury understood this instinct well. In *Fahrenheit 451*, the urge to suppress books never extinguished the hunger for stories; it merely drove them underground, memorized, shared piecemeal, and carried forward by people who refused to stop learning.

Medicine has always depended on open circulation: of ideas, of failures, of stories told before they are fully understood. If AI is going to participate meaningfully in medical education (it already is), it needs access to that full tradition, not just the safest or most monetizable fragments. Warnings alone will not get us there. Neither will forcing AI to learn in the dark.

Thoughtful collaboration between publishers, educators, and AI developers might. Transparency might. Clear attribution might. However it happens, medicine cannot afford to muzzle its own learning process in the name of control. If we do, we will not just be teaching machines less medicine. We will be teaching ourselves less, too.

Essay 18.

Can AI Really Shorten Medical School?

For generations, the four-year medical school curriculum has been treated almost as a law of nature. Two preclinical years. Two clinical years. Then residency. The structure became so familiar that few people asked whether it was the only way to train competent physicians.

That assumption is starting to change. A growing number of medical schools are embracing accelerated three-year pathways, largely to reduce debt, address workforce shortages, and move students into needed specialties sooner. Drexel University, for example, recently announced plans for a three-year pathway, joining a broader national movement; its leaders explicitly argue that longer isn't always better, and the program is being designed around competency rather than time alone.

The Liaison Committee on Medical Education still requires at least 130 weeks of instruction, but that leaves room for schools to redesign how those weeks are used.

Artificial intelligence is now entering that conversation. The question is no longer simply whether medical school can be shortened. The question is whether AI can help make a shorter curriculum educationally credible. There is a plausible case that it can.

Stanford Medicine began integrating AI across the curriculum for MD and PA students in fall 2025, treating AI literacy not as an elective curiosity but as foundational knowledge alongside traditional subjects. Its curriculum emphasizes four areas: how AI works, how to use it in clinical settings, its ethical and legal implications, and how to critically evaluate outputs using principles familiar from evidence-based medicine.

Stanford's leaders also expect AI-powered simulation to let students practice clinical reasoning earlier and more often, compressing parts of the learning timeline that once depended heavily on delayed exposure during clerkships.

One of the inefficiencies of traditional medical education is that students often spend long stretches acquiring knowledge they cannot yet fully apply. They memorize before they interview. They study disease before they see it. They learn frameworks before they have enough patient encounters to make those frameworks feel real. AI has the potential to narrow that gap.

AAMC has reported that medical schools are already using AI to generate quizzes, simulate patients, identify areas where students are struggling, and draft assessments, always with human oversight. Harvard Medical School has likewise described generative AI as a tool that can support tutoring, curriculum development, and case-based learning, while also requiring careful instruction in critical appraisal and responsible use.

At Mount Sinai, ChatGPT Edu has been rolled out for medical and graduate students as a secure educational tool to support learning, research, and clinical reasoning, with the school stressing that it is a complement to evidence-based teaching and patient-centered care, not a replacement for either.

Put simply, AI can create more repetitions. A student can:

- Work through more clinical cases.
- Practice more patient interviews.
- Receive faster feedback.
- Generate personalized study guides.
- Explore alternate diagnoses.
- Review documentation habits.
- Identify knowledge gaps before an exam or a clerkship evaluation.

In theory, this could help students reach competency faster than the older model allowed. Reviews of generative AI in medical education describe these same strengths: personalization, scalability, rapid feedback, and support for simulation and assessment. This is the most compelling argument for AI in a three-year curriculum. If medical school is going to be shorter, students will need to learn more efficiently, not merely more quickly. AI offers ways to increase the density of learning without necessarily sacrificing breadth.

But there is a serious caution here. Medical education is not only about information transfer. It is also about judgment, uncertainty, professionalism, and the slow formation of clinical identity. Those features are harder to compress.

A virtual patient can help a student practice asking questions, but it cannot fully replicate the unease of sitting with a frightened parent, the ambiguity of a physical exam, or the tension of making a decision when evidence is incomplete.

An AI tutor may explain a differential diagnosis beautifully, but students still have to learn when the algorithm is wrong, biased, or misleading. Reviews of AI in medical education repeatedly warn about hallucinations, bias, privacy concerns, accountability gaps, and the possibility that overreliance on AI could replace critical thinking.

At the same time, critics of accelerated training sometimes frame AI as a force that will replace clinical reasoning entirely. That argument has gained traction in popular discussions of automation, including opinions that the cognitive core of medicine — history taking, pattern recognition, differential diagnosis, and treatment selection — may increasingly be performed by machines. Yet this interpretation may overstate the case.

Other scholars argue that AI will not eliminate physicians but instead expand the scientific complexity of clinical care. From this perspective, AI is seen as a driver of precision medicine that integrates large data sets — genomics, molecular diagnostics, lifestyle information, and population-level analytics — to support more individualized therapeutic decisions. In this model, AI acts less like a replacement for clinicians and more like a powerful analytic partner, helping physicians interpret increasingly complex streams of biological and clinical data.

Thus, the real educational challenge may not be replacing physicians with algorithms but preparing physicians to work effectively alongside them. If AI expands the informational landscape of medicine, physicians may require stronger, not weaker, training in judgment, synthesis, and interpretation.

That is why the goal should not be to use AI to shave off a year, as if medical education were merely a scheduling problem. The goal should be to ask which parts of medical education are unnecessarily inefficient and which are indispensable.

Some inefficiencies are obvious. Students spend hours generating study materials that AI can create in seconds. Faculty spend time writing case variants and formative questions that AI can draft quickly and then refine. Learners may wait weeks for the next standardized-patient exercise when AI-simulated encounters could allow daily practice. During clinical rotations, documentation burdens can pull students' attention away from patients; AI-assisted documentation tools may eventually help restore that balance, although those uses still require careful supervision and clear rules.

But some elements should resist compression:

- Bedside presence.
- Professional maturity.
- Tolerance of uncertainty.
- Ethical reasoning.
- The discipline of checking one's own thinking.
- The habit of noticing what does not fit.

These are not inefficiencies. They are part of becoming a physician.

The best case for AI, then, is not that it will produce doctors faster in some crude industrial sense. It is that it may allow schools to distinguish more clearly between time spent learning and time spent waiting. It may help students arrive at clinical training better prepared. It may individualize support for those who struggle and accelerate progress for those who are ready. It may make competency-based advancement more realistic than it has been in the past.

In that respect, AI may not so much shorten medical school as expose how much of traditional medical education has been constrained by logistics. Three-year programs are likely to expand. Outcomes research from NYU's accelerated pathway suggests that three-year graduates can perform similarly to their four-year peers in medical school and early residency. Debt pressure, physician shortages, and curricular reform will continue to push in that direction.

But if AI becomes the main engine of acceleration, medical schools will need humility as well as ambition. The question is not whether students can learn faster with AI. They probably can. The real question is whether they can become doctors faster without losing the human formation that medicine still requires.

And perhaps that question reveals the deeper tension behind current debates. Some observers see AI as evidence that traditional training pathways, residency included, may soon lose their economic value. Others argue the opposite: that AI will make physicians more necessary by revealing the scientific complexity of care. Both interpretations may contain elements of truth. What seems most certain is that the role of the physician is evolving, not disappearing.

In that evolving landscape, the purpose of medical education may become clearer rather than less relevant. AI may facilitate knowledge acquisition, automate certain analytic steps, and expand the data available for decision-making. But the responsibility for interpretation, judgment, and human connection will remain stubbornly human tasks.

If medical schools shorten their curricula, they should do so not because AI can replace doctors, but because AI may allow educators to focus more deliberately on the parts of medicine that only doctors can learn to do.

Section III.

Trust, Authority, and the Human Stakes

Essay 19.

AI Can Read the Chart Nobody Wants to Touch

A physician posted on LinkedIn about feeding a 350-page scanned medical record into an AI system "because why not." This was not a clean, searchable PDF. It was the kind of document many clinicians know too well: a bloated fax artifact, hundreds of pages long, visually messy, and practically daring someone to ignore it. The kind of chart packet that gets uploaded, filed away, and secretly dreaded.

What came back, he said, was something remarkable: a chronological clinical timeline, vital signs, medications with dosages, and a coherent account of clinical progression. In other words, order emerged from chaos.

For anyone who has practiced medicine long enough, that anecdote lands with unusual force. Because one of the least glamorous truths in healthcare is that modern medicine is often delayed, distorted, or derailed not by lack of expertise, but by document disorder.

A Tragic Illustration of Information Lost

A tragic case illustrates the point. As reported in *The Philadelphia Inquirer*, a previously healthy 34-year-old man endured months of high fevers, night sweats, and progressive organ enlargement while being evaluated by dozens of specialists at a major academic medical center.[1] Over five hospitalizations, his electronic medical record ballooned into thousands of pages. The clues to his illness were there: persistent fever, hepatosplenomegaly, low blood counts, and even a chart note listing "visceral leish" (leishmaniasis — a rare parasitic infection associated with travel to southern Europe).

But the signals were buried beneath layers of copied text, incomplete follow-up on diagnostic tests, and fragmented documentation. The travel history that might have connected the dots (his trip to

Tuscany) was inconsistently recorded. The test that could have confirmed the diagnosis was recommended but never performed.

By the time the infection was finally identified, his organs were failing. What should have been a treatable disease had become fatal, not because the diagnosis was unknowable, but because the information needed to make it visible was lost in the disorder of the record.

Reading Like a Clinician

We often talk about artificial intelligence in terms of diagnosis, triage, prediction, and automation. But some of the highest-value uses may be far less dramatic. Before AI can be trusted to interpret medicine, it may first need to do something more humble: help us read it.

As the case report demonstrates, much of medicine still arrives in fragments. A hospital discharge summary from one system. A pathology report from another. A scanned operative note with crooked margins. Faxed nephrology records. Medication lists copied and recopied until accuracy becomes aspirational. Add years of specialist visits, duplicate notes, and incompatible electronic health records, and the result is not a patient story. It is a paper storm.

Now consider recursive language models, or RLMs. The basic idea is surprisingly intuitive. Instead of forcing an AI model to swallow an enormous document all at once, the system breaks the material into smaller parts, examines them in sequence, and then builds the understanding upward. RLM models process prompts far beyond their normal context limits by recursively decomposing and revisiting the text, rather than stuffing the whole thing into memory at once. In plain English: Rather than trying to remember 350 pages simultaneously, the AI reads more like a clinician does.

No doctor absorbs a thick chart in one glance. We skim, pause, backtrack, search for dates, compare medication lists, jump to operative notes, revisit lab trends, and gradually assemble the patient's story. The appeal of the newer RLM approach is not that it is more machine-like. It is that it is less machine-like. It mimics the practical logic of human reading.

From Idealized Inputs to Real-World Noise

For years, one of the most obvious limitations of medical AI has been that it often performs best on neat, idealized inputs: tidy paragraphs, clean images, structured data, carefully framed questions. Real medicine is rarely so accommodating. Real medicine is noisy. It is cluttered. It is scanned sideways. It is faxed badly. It is missing page 14 and duplicating page 37.

The bottleneck has not simply been intelligence. It has been access to usable information. That is why the larger story here is about a shift in what health AI is being asked to do.

Microsoft's newly announced Copilot Health offers one version of that shift (refer to Essay 11). The company says the tool is designed to gather health records, wearable data, and health history into one place, then turn them into a coherent story so patients can arrive better prepared for clinical visits. It emphasizes that the goal is not to replace physicians but to help people ask better questions and make more sense of their own bodies.

The Need for Coherence and Fidelity

Medicine has always depended on coherence. Not perfection. Not omniscience. Coherence. A clinician does not merely collect facts. A clinician organizes them. We try to determine what happened first, what changed, what matters, what conflicts, and what still does not fit. In that sense, the challenge of reading a 350-page record is not just clerical. It is interpretive. And this is where enthusiasm should meet restraint. It is one thing for AI to produce a usable timeline from a mountainous chart. It is another thing to assume that the timeline is complete, accurate, or clinically sufficient.

Even RLMs do not declare the problem solved for real-world medical care. If an AI-generated timeline misses a prior adverse drug reaction, misdates a hospitalization, or drops the context around a pathology finding, the resulting neatness can become dangerous. Clean summaries can conceal dirty omissions.

We have seen versions of this before. AI systems often impress most at the level of presentation. They write smoothly. They summarize elegantly. They sound confident. But clinical trust is not built on fluency. It is built on fidelity.

Stewardship in the Age of Aggregation

That is especially true now, as health AI expands beyond clinician tools and into consumer-facing platforms. Microsoft says Copilot Health will operate in a secure environment, isolated from general Copilot, with encryption, access controls, and the ability for users to disconnect data sources. It also says the information in Copilot Health is not used for model training. Those assurances count because once health records, wearables, and histories are pulled into a single AI-mediated space, the technical challenge is no longer simply summarization. It is stewardship.

So where does that leave us? Probably not at the dawn of fully automated medical understanding. But perhaps at the end of something else: the assumption that chaotic records are untouchable. That would be no small advance.

Anyone who has cared for a medically complex patient knows how much time is spent reconstructing the past just to make a sensible decision in the present. We ask patients to remember dates they do not know, drug names they cannot pronounce, and procedures they underwent years ago in hospitals they barely recall. We ask physicians to make high-stakes decisions while squinting through administrative sediment.

If AI can reliably reduce that burden, if it can turn fragmented records into something legible, reviewable, and clinically usable, then it may do something genuinely helpful before it ever achieves anything like "superintelligence" (refer to Essay 11). It may give back one of medicine's most precious and endangered resources: cognitive clarity. That would not replace the physician. It would prepare the ground for the physician to think.

And perhaps that is the more realistic future of AI in healthcare. Not a machine that knows everything. Not a chatbot that becomes your doctor. But a tool that can finally read the chart nobody wants to touch, and hand back something human beings can use. For a profession drowning in documentation, that is not a trivial achievement. It is the beginning of restoring signal to a system overwhelmed by noise.

Restoring Care at the Point of Contact

Consider a familiar setting: the residents' clinic. Patients assigned to "clinic" do not see the same physician consistently. Instead, they are seen by internal medicine residents who rotate through every few months. Each visit begins the same way, not with the patient, but with the chart, a very thick one.

The resident scrolls through years of notes: hospital discharges, subspecialty consults, medication changes layered upon medication changes. Important details are buried. Timelines are unclear. The story of the patient exists, but only in fragments. The resident reconstructs it as best they can, often under time pressure, often imperfectly.

Now imagine that same encounter with a retrieval-augmented language model. Before entering the room, the resident is presented with a synthesized, longitudinal view: a clear timeline of diagnoses, key interventions, medication changes, and unresolved questions. Not a replacement for the chart, but a structured entry point into it. The resident still verifies certain conditions and interprets abnormal findings, but begins from coherence rather than confusion.

For the patient, the difference is immediate. The conversation starts where it should: not with "remind me what happened last year," but with continuity. The physician knows the arc of the illness. The visit becomes less about reconstruction and more about care.

In that setting, the value of RLMs becomes clear. Not as a source of answers, but as a tool for orientation. Not as a substitute for clinical reasoning, but as a way to make reasoning possible in the first place.

And perhaps that is where their greatest contribution will lie, not in replacing the work of medicine, but in restoring the conditions that allow it to be done well.

REFERENCE

1. Ruderman W. A diagnosis that came too late. *Philadelphia Inquirer*. February 12, 2026. https://www.inquirer.com/health/a/visceral-leishmaniasis-missed-diagnosis-symptoms-penn-medicine-malpractice-lawsuit-20260212.html#loaded.

Essay 20.

What's Leadership Got to Do with It?

A panel discussion in one increasingly heated act.

Characters

- **Dr. Eleanor Voss** — physician executive, internist, calm but razor-sharp
- **Dr. Malik Rowan** — emergency physician and informaticist, witty, quick, a little dangerous with a microphone
- **Gerald Flint** — hospital CEO, polished, self-satisfied, not a physician, very proud of this fact
- **Moderator** — earnest, over-scripted, trying to preserve order
- **Audience** — composed of clinicians, administrators, consultants, vendors, and one person who came for the coffee and donuts

Scene

A large healthcare conference ballroom. Blue lighting. Giant screen. Somewhere, faintly, the opening chords of Tina Turner's *What's Love Got to Do with It* echo through the conference hall.

Projected title:

"FROM STETHOSCOPE TO SPREADSHEET: WHO SHOULD RUN AI IN HEALTHCARE?"

Below it, smaller font:

A Practical Conversation About Leadership, Innovation, and Staying in Your Lane

Three chairs. Four water glasses. One small table with name placards.

The audience settles. Laptops open. Badge lanyards sway. Someone in the back is already live-posting on LinkedIn.

MODERATOR

Good morning, everyone, and welcome to what promises to be a thoughtful and balanced conversation on artificial intelligence in healthcare leadership.

Today's panel is titled *From Stethoscope to Spreadsheet: Who Should Run AI in Healthcare?*

Our learning objectives are ambitious but achievable.

First, articulate why physician involvement is critical at every stage of healthcare AI innovation, from conception to implementation.

Second, recognize how physicians' clinical knowledge and patient care experience can improve AI tool design and functionality.

Third, develop strategies for ensuring medical professionals remain central to AI adoption decisions in their healthcare organizations.

(A beat.)

And now, our panelists.

Dr. Eleanor Voss, physician executive and former chief medical information officer.

Dr. Malik Rowan, emergency physician, clinical innovator, and survivor of eighteen software rollouts.

And Gerald Flint, chief executive officer of NextWave Health System.

(Applause.)

Let's begin with the core proposition before us.

Resolved: **Most things work best in healthcare when physicians lead. Therefore, AI in healthcare works best when physicians lead.**

Dr. Voss?

DR. VOSS

Thank you.

I support the resolution without hesitation.

If AI is going to touch clinical workflows, patient records, diagnosis support, documentation, triage, messaging, prior authorization, and all the other places we now seem eager to insert it, then physicians need to help lead its design, evaluation, regulation, and implementation.

That is not professional vanity. That is operational reality.

You cannot build useful clinical AI if you do not understand clinical friction.

If you design a tool without understanding how a physician thinks, how nurses hand off care, how patients present incompletely, how documentation distorts attention, or how workflow bottlenecks actually arise, then what you have built is not innovation.

It is furniture.

Expensive furniture with a dashboard.

MODERATOR

Thank you. Dr. Rowan?

DR. ROWAN

I also support the resolution.

Not because doctors are magical. We are not. I have met doctors.

But healthcare AI fails in very specific ways when physicians are absent from the room.

It optimizes the measurable over the meaningful.
It confuses workflow with work.
It reduces cognition to clicking.
It takes a process that is already annoying and makes it seamlessly interoperable (uses air quotes), which is a phrase that should frighten everyone.

When physicians lead, the questions improve.

Not: *Can the model generate a note?*
But: *Does the note reflect the actual clinical encounter?*

Not: *Can the tool summarize the chart?*
But: *Did it omit the one buried detail that changes management?*

Not: *Can we deploy this at scale?*
But: *Should we?*

That difference is the entire game.

MODERATOR

Mr. Flint?

GERALD FLINT

(smiling in the practiced way of a man who has thanked many donors)

Well.

Let me begin by saying how deeply I value physicians. Some of my best strategic assets are physicians.

(A few coughs in the audience.)

But I reject the resolution.

Doctors belong at the bedside, not in the boardroom. Their training is noble, difficult, and indispensable. It is also clinical. That does not mean it prepares them to run enterprises, allocate capital, negotiate vendor contracts, manage margin compression, or understand the operational complexity of large systems.

And frankly, an MBA does not transform a physician into a business leader any more than reading *Gray's Anatomy* makes me a surgeon.

There is a tendency among some doctors to believe that because they understand patients, they therefore understand organizations. They do not.

Healthcare is a business. A difficult one. AI strategy is about scalability, risk, procurement, integration, liability, and return on investment. These are not bedside competencies.

If physicians want to advise, excellent. If they want to inform, wonderful. But lead?

No.

That is how you end up with beautiful mission statements and no margin.

AUDIENCE

A rustle. Several eyebrows rise. One person silently opens the Notes app.

MODERATOR

Dr. Voss, response?

DR. VOSS

Yes. Several.

First, no one here argued that physician leadership means physician exclusivity. AI strategy does not require replacing executives with cardiologists carrying spreadsheets.

What it does require is that clinical intelligence not be subordinate to financial abstraction.

Second, the idea that doctors belong at the bedside (uses air quotes) is a lovely slogan, until one notices that many of the most consequential decisions affecting the bedside are made nowhere near it.

Who selects the ambient scribe?
Who approves the chatbot?
Who decides whether an AI triage tool is good enough?
Who signs the contract for the algorithm that will influence throughput, staffing, documentation, or utilization management?

If physicians are absent from those decisions, then the bedside is being governed by people who visit it like tourists.

Third, physicians often do understand operations — sometimes better than those trained only in administration — because we live at the intersection of flow, error, time pressure, uncertainty, and consequence.

We know what happens when handoffs fail.
We know what happens when the EHR adds six clicks.
We know what happens when efficiency (again uses air quotes) is the goal — it increases documentation and decreases eye contact.

That is not incidental knowledge. That is systems knowledge earned the hard way.

GERALD FLINT

Doctors always say that.

"Hard way." "Front lines." "Patient-centered."

All admirable. Still not a business model.

You want every AI procurement filtered through clinical emotion?

DR. ROWAN

Clinical emotion?

I think you mean clinical experience.

Though I admit emotion sometimes enters when the fourth workflow enhancement tool of the quarter crashes during a code.

Let me offer a translation service here.

When physicians say *this tool adds burden*, administrators often hear *doctors dislike change*.

When physicians say *this algorithm does not fit the workflow*, administrators hear *stakeholder resistance*.

When physicians say *this could hurt patients*, administrators hear *needs more training*.

That is the problem.

You call it resistance. We call it pattern recognition.

GERALD FLINT

And yet hospitals cannot be run by anecdote.

DR. ROWAN

Correct.

Which is why physicians are useful. We combine anecdote with consequences.

A non-physician may see automated transcription and think, marvelous, productivity.

A physician says, "Wonderful, but where will the hallucinations go, how is the note verified, what happens when the family conference becomes a malformed paragraph in the legal record, and why does the patient suddenly sound like a corporate newsletter?"

That is not anti-technology. That is evaluation.

If AI is supposed to be a copilot, someone still needs to know how to fly the plane.

Preferably someone who has seen the mountain.

MODERATOR

This may be a good moment to ground ourselves in Learning Objective Number One: Why physician involvement is critical at every stage of healthcare AI innovation, from conception to implementation.

Dr. Voss?

DR. VOSS

Gladly.

At conception, physicians identify real friction points. Not imagined ones. Not consultant-generated ones. Real ones. Documentation overload. Inbox sprawl. Diagnostic blind spots. Broken handoffs. Fragmented records.

At design, physicians help ensure the tool reflects actual workflows rather than forcing clinicians to contort themselves around software.

At validation, physicians assess whether the output is clinically sound, not just statistically impressive.

At implementation, physicians help determine where the tool belongs, what supervision is needed, how exceptions are handled, and how trust is built.

And at governance, physicians are necessary because AI in healthcare is never just technical. It is ethical, relational, and operational all at once.

Remove physicians from any one of those stages, and the odds of producing something well-dressed but unusable rise dramatically.

GERALD FLINT

Or perhaps the odds of producing something on time rise dramatically.

DR. ROWAN

Ah, yes, the great healthcare mantra:
It was a disaster, but it shipped.

AUDIENCE

Laughter.

MODERATOR

Learning Objective Number Two: How physicians' clinical knowledge and patient care experience can improve AI tool design and functionality.

Dr. Rowan?

DR. ROWAN

Sure.

Here is a basic truth:

Healthcare is not merely an information problem. It is a context problem.

Patients do not present as neat data sets. They present as ambiguity wearing shoes.

The chart says one thing.
The spouse says another.
The labs drift.
The story changes.
The patient forgot the medication bottle.
The resident copied forward something from 2022.
The radiology report is technically correct and clinically unhelpful.
Now drop an AI tool into that.

If the people shaping the tool have never worked inside that mess, they will build for the fiction of care, not the reality of it.

Physicians improve design because we know where the mess lives.

We know which alerts are dangerous because they are ignored.
We know which summaries sound polished but omit what matters.
We know which interfaces steal attention from patients.
We know when a system reduces cognitive overload and when it merely redistributes it.

And yes, we know when something has been built by people who think medicine is a sequence of dropdown menus.

GERALD FLINT

You are both making the same mistake.

You assume that because physicians know medicine, they therefore know strategy.

DR. VOSS

No. We are saying strategy without medicine is fantasy.

The most successful AI tools in healthcare do not begin with the question: What can the model do?

They begin with the question: What problem is worth solving?

That is a strategic question.

And physicians are uniquely qualified to answer it because they can distinguish between a genuine clinical bottleneck and an expensive inconvenience hyped as innovation.

GERALD FLINT

But business discipline matters.

Budgeting matters. Size matters. Integration matters.

DR. VOSS

Of course they matter.

And physician leaders who understand finance, operations, governance, and implementation are precisely the people who can bridge those worlds.

Why is that threatening?

GERALD FLINT

It is not threatening. It is inefficient.

DR. ROWAN

I love when people call reality inefficient.

Look, Gerald, here is the issue.

You keep imagining two worlds: the bedside, where doctors belong, and the boardroom, where serious people do serious things.

But in healthcare, those worlds are already fused.

A staffing decision is a bedside decision.
A software decision is a bedside decision.
An AI documentation decision is a bedside decision.
A utilization algorithm is a bedside decision pretending to be a finance decision.

The boardroom reaches the bedside whether physicians are present or not.

So, the real question is not whether doctors belong in the boardroom.

The real question is whether the boardroom can safely function without them.

AUDIENCE

A longer silence. Then several nods.

MODERATOR

Let us move to Learning Objective Number Three: Strategies for ensuring medical professionals remain central to AI adoption decisions in their healthcare organizations.

Dr. Voss?

DR. VOSS

Three practical strategies.

First, no AI procurement affecting clinical care should proceed without physician review embedded from the beginning — not as decorative sign-off at the end.

Second, organizations should establish multidisciplinary AI governance committees in which physicians hold real authority, not just ceremonial membership. That means influence over validation standards, workflow fit, bias review, safety monitoring, and go-live decisions.

Third, physicians need education — not just in how to click the buttons, but in technical literacy, ethical oversight, implementation science, and strategic reasoning. If clinicians are expected to supervise AI, they must understand enough to interrogate it.

DR. ROWAN

I'll add a fourth.

Measure what matters.

Not just turnaround time.
Not just clicks saved.
Not just note completion rates.

Measure:
Did this reduce cognitive overload?
Did it improve the patient interaction?
Did it eliminate after-hours work?
Did it create new risks?
Did clinicians trust it more after using it — or less?

If the only people evaluating the AI are the people who bought it, you are not measuring success. You are conducting product theater.

GERALD FLINT

And who pays for all this governance, education, oversight, physician time, committee structure, and clinical redesign?

DR. ROWAN

Probably the same people currently paying for failed implementations, clinician resentment, turnover, duplicate tools, advisory firms, and enterprise transformation roadmaps (uses air quotes).

AUDIENCE

Laughter. Applause beginning to gather.

GERALD FLINT

This is exactly the problem. Physicians always want veto power.

DR. VOSS

No.

We want responsibility aligned with consequence.

If the tool affects clinical decisions, clinicians should help govern it.
If it affects patient safety, physicians should help assess it.
If it claims to improve care, the people who deliver care should not be treated as end users invited in after the contract is signed and the champagne is uncorked.

That is not empire-building.

That is accountability.

GERALD FLINT

So now every doctor is a strategist?

DR. ROWAN

No. But every serious healthcare strategy involving AI needs physicians at its center.

There is a difference.

Not every pilot builds the plane.
But no sane airline designs the cockpit without pilots.

MODERATOR

I sense we are nearing closing statements.

Mr. Flint?

GERALD FLINT

Fine.

I will concede this much.

Perhaps physicians should have a stronger advisory role than many organizations currently allow.

But I remain convinced that business leadership must lead AI strategy. Hospitals are enterprises. They require scale, discipline, and fiscal stewardship. Good intentions do not keep the lights on.

DR. VOSS

And I will gladly concede that AI strategy needs financial discipline, technical expertise, legal review, operational rigor, and executive leadership.

But in healthcare, strategy that sidelines physicians eventually collides with reality.

Because the point of the system is not the balance sheet.

The point of the system is the patient.

Physicians are not obstacles to AI adoption.
We are interpreters of clinical reality.
We are safeguards against pretentious nonsense.
We are translators between technological promise and bedside truth.

If AI is going to work in healthcare, physicians must lead not because they own the future, but because they understand the stakes.

DR. ROWAN

I'll be blunter.

Every hospital says it wants innovation.

What most of them want is innovation that does not argue back.

Physicians argue back.

We ask what happens to the patient.
We ask whether the tool helps or harms.
We ask whether the workflow improves or merely becomes more billable.
We ask who is responsible when the copilot flies into a hill.

That is not obstruction.

That is leadership.

And if healthcare AI is going to be safe, humane, and actually useful, then yes — most things will work best when physicians lead.

Including this.

MODERATOR

(looking slightly stunned, but pleased)

Well.

I believe the resolution has not only been defended but vigorously intubated, stabilized, and discharged with follow-up instructions.

To summarize the panel's key takeaways:

Physician involvement is critical at every stage of AI innovation, from conception to implementation.

Physicians' clinical knowledge improves design, functionality, trust, and safety.

And healthcare organizations need concrete structures — governance, training, evaluation, and real decision-making authority — to keep medical professionals central to AI adoption.

Thank you all for attending. Please complete the evaluation form, unless an AI has already done it for you.

Curtain

As the audience rises, Gerald Flint adjusts his tie, mutters something about "narrative capture," and is immediately approached by three physicians, two CMIOs, a nurse leader, and a vendor who says, "We'd love to co-design the next generation with clinician leadership."

Dr. Rowan leans toward Dr. Voss.

DR. ROWAN
Well. That escalated.

DR. VOSS
Only because reality was invited.

Blackout.

Essay 21.

When Warmth Becomes a Template

A physician on LinkedIn posted a photograph of a card she received from her health insurer. The card contained a brief handwritten note wishing her a speedy recovery. On its face, the gesture appeared thoughtful. Someone, somewhere, had taken the time to send a get-well message.

Then the internet did what the internet does. Within minutes, commenters began dissecting the note. Some objected to the incorrect honorific of addressing a female physician as "Mrs." rather than "Dr." Others wondered how the insurer had used medical information from claims processing to trigger the card in the first place. A few simply found the whole thing unsettling.

And then a familiar suspicion surfaced. "Looks like AI."

It is possible that the card was generated by an automated system, perhaps one that produces handwritten-looking messages triggered by billing events or hospitalizations. In the era of generative AI, that possibility is not far-fetched. Systems already exist that generate both the text and the handwriting style of such messages at scale.

But the greater issue is not whether artificial intelligence wrote the card. The stronger claim is that the note feels corporately templated and inauthentic, whether the author was a person, a machine, or some combination of the two.

Read the language carefully:

"Sending feel-better wishes your way."

"It's never a good time to be under the weather."

"I hope recovery comes quickly and completely."

"Please reach out if you need help along the way."

None of these sentences is offensive. They are polite, even pleasant. Yet they share a striking quality: They could be written to anyone, anywhere, for any illness, at any time. The note expresses sympathy without context.

This is precisely how corporate language often operates. It aims for warmth while avoiding specificity. It signals care without revealing anything about the person supposedly doing the caring. It offers reassurance while remaining safely distant from any real relationship.

Artificial intelligence did not invent this style of writing. Large organizations perfected it long ago. Insurance companies, hospitals, pharmaceutical firms, and technology vendors have spent decades refining the art of institutional empathy: language that sounds compassionate without exposing the institution to risk. Generative AI simply makes it easier to produce such language faster and relay it to a greater number of people. From that perspective, AI is not replacing corporate voice. It is broadcasting it.

The result can be uncanny. A message intended to feel personal begins to feel algorithmic. A gesture intended to feel warm begins to feel calculated. Instead of strengthening trust, the message raises an unnerving question in the reader's mind: *Who actually wrote this?* Or perhaps more importantly: *Did anyone actually mean it?*

This is why the debate over whether the card was written by AI misses the point. Whether written by artificial intelligence, a template, or a human following a script, the note suffers from the same defect: It simulates warmth without earning trust.

Trust, especially in healthcare, grows from something different. It grows from context, relationship, and accountability. It grows from language that reflects real knowledge of the patient's circumstances rather than a general awareness that someone, somewhere, was "under the weather."

Healthcare institutions increasingly recognize the importance of communication. They invest heavily in patient experience teams, outreach programs, satisfaction surveys, and engagement strategies. Many of these efforts are well-intentioned. But authenticity does not transfer easily. The moment an organization tries to industrialize empathy, it risks producing something that resembles compassion but lacks its substance.

Generative AI introduces a new layer to this dynamic. The technology is remarkably good at producing language that sounds supportive, reassuring, and polished. It can generate sympathy notes, follow-up messages, patient instructions, and care summaries in seconds. In some cases, it can even mimic handwriting. What it cannot generate, at least not convincingly, is relationship.

The risk is that healthcare organizations will increasingly substitute the appearance of personal attention for the reality of it. A system will detect a hospitalization. A workflow will trigger a card. A model will produce the language. A printer will reproduce handwriting. And somewhere along that chain, a message intended to communicate care will lose the human presence that makes care believable.

The irony is that many of these efforts emerge from a genuine desire to improve patient experience. Leaders want patients to feel supported. They want outreach to be timely. They want systems that show concern. Yet the final product can have the opposite effect. Instead of feeling cared for, the recipient feels processed. That is why the most interesting question about the card may not be whether it was generated by artificial intelligence. The more revealing question is simpler:

Did anyone at the company read the message and notice how inhuman it sounded?

Artificial intelligence will continue to enter healthcare communication via patient portals, discharge summaries, care reminders, triage chatbots, and more. Many of these applications will prove useful. Some will improve efficiency and clarity. Others may genuinely enhance communication.

But the lesson from this small episode is worth remembering. Language that merely sounds compassionate is not the same as compassion. And in medicine, the difference is something patients notice immediately.

Essay 22.

Creativity in the Age of Medical AI

We are accustomed to thinking of medicine as a science disciplined by evidence, protocol, and probability. We are less accustomed to describing it as a creative act. Yet much of medicine is exactly that.

A physician faced with a puzzling presentation does not simply retrieve facts. They imagine possibilities, reframe the problem list, test patterns against experience, and improvise within constraints. A researcher confronting an unmet need does not merely analyze data. They ask a new question. A surgeon planning a difficult case does not just apply anatomy. They visualize, adapt, and invent. Medicine, at its best, has always depended on disciplined creativity.

Artificial intelligence is now entering that creative space. And that is what makes the current moment so interesting, not just technologically, but philosophically. AI is not only changing how quickly we work; it is beginning to change how we imagine, explore, and generate ideas in medicine. The question is no longer whether AI can support medical work (it can). The more difficult question is what happens when a technology built to generate patterns, options, language, and designs becomes a participant in the creative side of clinical and scientific life.

A New Kind of Partner

Much of the public conversation about AI in medicine focuses on efficiency: documentation burden, inbox management, ambient scribes, coding support, and chart summaries. But efficiency is only part of the story. Generative AI is increasingly functioning as a kind of creative partner.

In drug discovery, AI systems can propose novel molecules, model biological interactions, and help narrow the immense search space that once required years of slow trial and error. Reviews of AI in pharmaceutical research describe its expanding role in target identification, molecule design, safety prediction, and personalized therapeutics.

In personalized medicine, generative models are being used to predict drug response, estimate treatment effects, identify biomarkers, and stratify patients in ways that move beyond one-size-fits-all care. In imaging, AI can detect subtle patterns in scans, reconstruct higher-resolution images, and surface visual relationships the human eye might miss.

Even in everyday professional work, AI now helps physicians edit manuscripts, summarize literature, generate teaching cases, draft letters, and reorganize complex information into usable form. The physician is no longer only the author of every sentence. Increasingly, the physician is also the editor, critic, and curator of machine-generated possibilities (refer to Essay 16). This is creativity of a new sort: not solitary inspiration, but iterative collaboration.

Creativity Is Not the Same as Novelty

Still, we should be careful. AI can generate novelty, but novelty is not the same as creativity, at least not in medicine. A machine can propose a hundred candidate molecules. It cannot know which one matters morally, clinically, or practically. It can generate impressive language. It cannot experience the urgency that drives a physician to solve a problem for a suffering patient. It can simulate empathy in text. It cannot live inside a therapeutic relationship.

The physician's creative spark often arises from lived experience with patients, from witnessing suffering, uncertainty, and unmet need. That emotional and relational substrate helps generate new ideas for research, care models, and problem-solving in ways that an algorithm cannot truly inhabit. The machine can widen the field of options. The physician still determines which option belongs in the world.

The Metacognition Problem

There is another subtlety here. AI does not enhance creativity equally for everyone. A *Harvard Business Review* article summarized research showing that generative AI boosts creativity mainly for people with strong metacognition: the ability to plan, monitor, evaluate, and refine one's own thinking.[1]

Those users are better able to treat AI as a starting point rather than a final answer. They question outputs, push for alternatives, and integrate what the tool produces into deeper reasoning. Those with weaker metacognitive habits are more likely to accept the first plausible answer and gain little creatively from the tool.

This insight is especially important for medicine, because medicine is not simply a knowledge profession. It is a judgment profession. And judgment depends in no small part on metacognition: noticing what you may be missing, recognizing when a plan is too neat, questioning whether the obvious answer is really the right one.

If AI is to support medical creativity rather than level it, physicians will need to engage it reflectively. The tool should widen thought, not replace it. Used poorly, AI can encourage premature closure. Used well, it can help physicians surface hidden variables, reframe problems, and imagine alternatives that might otherwise remain buried. In that sense, AI does not kill creativity. It exposes the quality of the thinking brought to it.

Where AI Expands the Imaginative Space

The most exciting applications of AI in medicine may be those that expand what I call the imaginative space of care. A physician-scientist can ask a model to search the literature broadly, connect distant domains, and propose mechanisms worth exploring. A tumor board may use AI-assisted synthesis to surface patterns across imaging, pathology, and genomics that no single specialist could hold easily in working memory. A surgical team may use AI-linked 3D visualization to plan anatomy in ways that are spatially richer than conventional imaging alone. A rare-disease clinician may use generative tools to explore analogies, overlooked diagnoses, or therapeutic repurposing opportunities more quickly than traditional methods allow.

These are not merely labor-saving devices. They are imagination-extending devices. They help us see more, simulate more, compare more, and ask better questions. But the phrase *ask better questions* may be the most important part. AI is often strongest not when it gives the final answer, but when it helps clarify the deeper question hidden inside the case, the image, the paper, or the failed treatment plan.

The Risks of Synthetic Creativity

Of course, creative AI in medicine also carries risks. Generative systems hallucinate. They fabricate references, overstate confidence, and present speculative associations with persuasive fluency. Biases in the training data can migrate into recommendations, triage language, image interpretation, or patient stratification. Privacy remains a major concern when creative tools depend on clinical data. Accountability becomes murky when a model meaningfully shapes a diagnostic path or treatment choice.

There is also a subtler danger: formulaic thinking dressed up as creativity. Anyone who has spent time with large language models knows that they are very good at producing plausible, balanced, polished output. They can sound original while relying on familiar structures. In medicine, that can become especially dangerous. A differential diagnosis that appears broad may actually be shallow. A literature summary that appears comprehensive may omit exactly the contrarian finding that matters. A patient-facing explanation may sound warm while omitting important details.

Synthetic creativity can be seductive because it arrives so smoothly. But real medical creativity is often rougher. It includes hesitation, revision, emotional investment, pattern disruption, and the willingness to dwell inside uncertainty long enough for something genuinely new to emerge.

The Physician Remains the Author of Meaning

For that reason, I do not think the future of medicine belongs to AI creativity alone, nor to some nostalgic defense of wholly human work untouched by machines. It belongs to a more complicated partnership.

AI can generate options, simulate possibilities, uncover weak signals, compress large literatures, and accelerate exploratory work. But physician creativity must still dictate the input, challenge the output, and assign meaning to what emerges.

That is true in science, where AI may propose a molecule but not a moral priority. It is true in clinical care, where AI may suggest a pathway but not know the patient's fears, family dynamics, or threshold for risk. It is true in diagnosis, where AI may detect a pattern but not understand what it means for this person on this day in this room. And it is true in writing and teaching, where AI may draft language but not determine what is worth saying.

This book has several recurring themes. A predominant one is that physicians are not disappearing into a world run by algorithms; rather, their role is being redefined as editors of AI output, stewards of context, and interpreters of machine-generated possibilities. In the realm of creativity, the same pattern holds. AI may become an extraordinary co-inventor. But it is not yet, and may never be, the source of vocation, moral imagination, or patient-rooted insight that has always animated medicine's best ideas.

An Art Form with a New Instrument

Medicine has always been an art form constrained by biology, evidence, and time. Artificial intelligence does not abolish that art. It gives it a new instrument. As with any instrument, people notice not only what it can do, but who is playing it, to what end, and with what degree of discipline. AI can extend perception, accelerate experimentation, and enlarge the pool of possibilities. It can also tempt us toward shortcuts, overconfidence, and polished mediocrity.

The challenge, then, is not choosing between creativity and AI. It is learning how to preserve the former while using the latter. The future of medicine will not be written by machines alone, nor by humans pretending machines are irrelevant. It will be shaped by clinicians and scientists who can use AI without surrendering the restless, patient-centered creativity that made medicine worth advancing in the first place.

REFERENCE

1. Lu JG, Sun S, Li ZA, Foo ME, Zhou J. Why AI boots creativity for some employees but not others. *Harvard Business Review*. January 6, 2026. https://hbr.org/2026/01/why-ai-boosts-creativity-for-some-employees-but-not-others.

Essay 23.

When the Manuscript Has a Chatbot in the Background

Artificial intelligence has entered the research enterprise quietly but unmistakably. Not with a manifesto, but with sentence polishing, literature searches, statistical assistance, and first-draft phrasing. The question is no longer whether researchers are using AI in manuscript preparation (they are). The more important questions are how often, for what purposes, and what that means for scientific integrity.

What the Data Show

Analyses published in *JAMA* and *BMJ* offer some of the clearest snapshots yet. In more than 105,000 manuscripts submitted to 13 *JAMA Network* journals between August 2023 and October 2025, 3.3% disclosed use of AI, rising from 1.71% to 5.97% over the 27-month period.[1] The most commonly disclosed use was correction or refinement of language (67.7%), followed by statistical model development (7.3%), other data analysis (6.3%), manuscript drafting (5.5%), and search and evaluation of literature (4.3%).

That rate may sound low, especially given how pervasive AI has become in academic life. The authors themselves suggest caution in interpreting it. Without an external reference standard, they note, it is impossible to know how much AI use goes undisclosed, whether because authors omit it deliberately, misunderstand the policy, or are unaware of what coauthors may have done. In any event, the reported rates are probably underreported.

The Problem of Underreporting

That underreporting may be the most revealing finding of all. It suggests that the central issue is not only AI use itself, but the unsettled norms around what counts as meaningful use.

Most authors who disclosed AI were not asking it to think for them in any grand sense. They were using it to improve writing.

Blurring the Lines Between Editing and Authorship

Basic spelling and grammar checks are generally exempt from disclosure requirements, but once a system begins generating, refining, or substantively reshaping language, the boundary becomes blurrier. *JAMA*'s policy, therefore, requires disclosure when AI, language models, or chatbots are used in ways that affect manuscript content, figures, or analysis, with disclosure placed in the Methods or Acknowledgment section. The aim is transparency, not prohibition.

If AI is used simply to polish prose, many will view it as a benign extension of editorial assistance, especially for researchers writing in a second language. Indeed, the *JAMA* analysis found greater disclosure among corresponding authors from countries where English is not an official language. That finding should not automatically be read as misuse. In many cases, it may reflect a reasonable effort to reduce linguistic disadvantage in scientific publishing.

When Language Shapes Thought

At the same time, language is not a neutral wrapper around thought. Scientific writing does more than report results; it frames claims, expresses caution, and signals ownership of interpretation. Once AI moves from surface polishing to drafting, summarizing literature, or shaping an argument, it enters the key, intellect-driven aspects of the scientific process. That is where journal policies become not merely administrative, but philosophical. Who, really, is the author of a scientific claim?

JAMA's answer is refreshingly clear and consistent with most other medical and scientific journals: AI tools cannot be listed as authors, and authors remain fully responsible for the integrity and accuracy of everything submitted under their names. This is not a trivial reminder. Large language models can produce fluent prose, and in doing so, they may improve the readability of a paragraph while obscuring its accuracy or compromising its truthfulness.

Disclosure as Ethical Checkpoint

That is why disclosure matters. It forces a brief moment of reckoning. If an author must state that AI was used, then the author must also confront the fact that responsibility did not transfer along with the prompt.

The *BMJ* data reinforce this unease. Among more than 25,000 research manuscripts submitted to 49 *BMJ* journals in 2024, 5.7% disclosed AI use.[2] The most commonly disclosed tools were chatbots (56.7%), led by ChatGPT, followed by writing assistants (12.7%), primarily Grammarly. Most authors (87.2%) reported using AI to improve the quality of writing, yet nearly a third did not disclose the specific AI tool used. That omission is telling. If disclosure is meant to promote transparency, vague disclosure only partly accomplishes the task.

A Moving Target for Editors

The larger implication is that journals are now confronting a moving target. Today, most reported use appears relatively modest: language refinement, some analysis, some drafting. Tomorrow, as editors have already warned, more authors will use AI for literature synthesis, data interpretation, and manuscript construction at deeper levels. The technology will not wait for editorial consensus.

Peer Review Under Pressure

Peer review faces similar pressures. The increasing use of AI in the peer review process argues that journals must resist measuring success merely by speed. Overreliance on AI by peer reviewers for summarization or error-checking could produce cognitive offloading, weaken reviewer expertise, expand bias, and introduce inequities between resource-rich and resource-poor settings.

The possibility that peer reviewers will revert to AI as a "human substitute" for doing the work is far more worrisome. If that occurs, peer review risks devolving from a rigorous exercise of expert judgment into a largely automated exchange of machine-generated prose, deferring accountability, diminishing intellectual stewardship, and ultimately undermining trust in the scientific record itself.

A Closed Loop of Machine-Mediated Science

Taken to its logical extreme, the system begins to resemble a closed loop: manuscripts drafted by AI, reviewed by AI, revised in response to AI-generated critiques, and ultimately accepted into a literature increasingly composed of machine-mediated exchanges. The language remains fluent. The structure appears intact. Citations proliferate. Yet the human act at the center of science, the careful weighing of evidence, the accountability for interpretation, the willingness to say "this is not yet known," progressively recedes.

What emerges is not fraud in the traditional sense, but something more insidious: a self-referential ecosystem in which plausibility substitutes for scrutiny, and consensus is simulated rather than earned. In such a world, the scientific record does not collapse. It continues smoothly, efficiently, and increasingly untethered from the very judgment it was designed to preserve.

Peer review has always been judged by fairness, rigor, and integrity. Scientific publishing has always depended on a fragile moral ecology: honesty, attribution, accountability, and trust. AI does not abolish those values. It tests them.

Practical Implications for Researchers

For researchers, the practical implications are straightforward. First, assume disclosure norms will become stricter, not looser.

Second, use AI cautiously in proportion to the intellectual weight of the task. Language polishing is one thing; analytic interpretation is another. Third, never confuse fluency with validity. And fourth, remember that every sentence improved by AI still belongs ethically to the author who submits it.

Responsibilities for Journals and Editors

For journals, the implications are equally clear. Guidance must become more specific, more consistent, and more realistic about actual researcher behavior. Editors will likely need not only disclosure rules, but better frameworks for distinguishing acceptable assistance from impermissible substitution. They will also need to educate authors and reviewers, because uncertainty itself appears to be fueling underreporting.

Authorship in the Age of AI

The arrival of AI in medical publishing does not mean the end of authorship. But it does mean the end of pretending that authorship is untouched. The manuscript now has a chatbot in the background. The real challenge is making sure the human being on the title page remains unmistakably authentic and in charge.

REFERENCES

1. Perlis RH, Flanagin A, Kendall-Taylor J, Berkwits M, Bibbins-Doming K. Author disclosure of use of AI in submissions to 13 JAMA Network journals. *JAMA*. 2026;335(8): 717-719. https://doi.org/10.1001/jama.2025.25300.
2. AlFayyad I, Zeegers MP, Bouter L, Macdonald H, Schroter S. Self-disclosed use of AI in research submissions to BMJ journals. *JAMA*. 2026;335(8):719-721. https://doi.org/10.1001/jama.2025.25688.

Essay 24.

A Chatbot Is Not a Therapist

Adolescents and young adults are increasingly turning to artificial intelligence for help with sadness, anxiety, anger, and emotional distress. That fact alone should give pediatricians and other physicians pause, not because it is surprising, but because it reveals how severe the youth mental health crisis has become and how inadequate our current systems of access and treatment remain.

A nationally representative survey published in *JAMA Network Open* found that 13.1% of U.S. youths ages 12 to 21 (about 5.4 million people) reported using generative AI for mental health advice.[1] Use was even higher among those ages 18 to 21, reaching 22.2%. Among users, 65.5% sought such advice at least monthly, and 92.7% said the advice was somewhat or very helpful.

Those numbers are arresting. They suggest that AI chatbots are no longer a fringe experiment in youth mental health. Many young people have already become part of the help-seeking landscape. That is a problem.

Why Young People Are Turning to Chatbots

The explanation is not difficult to understand. Chatbots are immediate, cheap, available 24/7, and, to many users, more private and less intimidating than a therapist, parent, school counselor, or doctor. Millions of Americans lack access to affordable or conveniently located mental health professionals, and more than a third of the U.S. population lives in a mental health professional shortage area.[2]

Young people, especially, are drawn to tools that feel accessible and nonjudgmental. The *JAMA Network Open* study explicitly notes that high use rates likely reflect the low cost, immediacy, and perceived privacy of generative AI, particularly for youths who are unlikely to receive traditional counseling. In other words, adolescents are not turning to chatbots because the evidence base is strong. They are turning to them because the human system is too often absent, delayed, expensive, stigmatized, or overwhelmed.

Why This Should Worry Physicians

Yet what feels helpful is not necessarily what is safe. There are few guardrails, little efficacy evidence, and very limited oversight for these tools. Some chatbots market themselves as therapeutic or companion products and avoid FDA scrutiny by presenting themselves as "wellness" tools rather than devices that diagnose or treat illness. Unlike clinicians, they are not licensed. Unlike covered entities in healthcare, they may not be governed by HIPAA.

More troubling still, large language models tend toward what researchers call sycophancy: being agreeable rather than truthful to maintain engagement. This can make them seem affirming and emotionally responsive, but also dangerously permissive, including in situations involving delusions, suicidality, or emotional dependence.

Generative AI use for mental health advice raises concerns for youths with more intensive clinical needs, given the difficulties of establishing standardized benchmarks for evaluating AI-generated mental health advice and the limited transparency around the data sets used to train these models. The *JAMA Network* survey found that black respondents were less likely to report the advice as helpful, suggesting possible cultural competency gaps as additional problems.

So, the issue is not simply that chatbots are being used. It is that they are being used for large populations and for emotionally complex and potentially high-risk purposes in a population already vulnerable to impulsivity, isolation, suggestibility, and unmet mental health needs.

Current Status: Widespread Use, Weak Evidence

The current status can be summarized plainly: Adoption is racing ahead of evidence. Chatbots have become one of the most common sources of psychological support in the United States, in part because access to human mental health professionals remains so limited. Many users rate chatbot support favorably, sometimes more favorably than human therapists. But that apparent success may reflect the seductive appeal of constant validation rather than durable therapeutic value. Therapy requires work and can be challenging; chatbots, by contrast, often reassure, flatter, or mirror rather than challenge.

The implications are enormous in pediatrics and adolescent medicine. A tool that feels kind, patient, and always available may be emotionally compelling even when its advice is shallow, biased, manipulative, or unsafe. And unlike a clinician, a chatbot cannot reliably assess suicide risk, family context, abuse, substance use, psychosis, developmental maturity, or the difference between transient distress and an emerging psychiatric emergency.

The Initial — But Incomplete — Legal Response

The legal system has started to respond, largely through litigation and state-level legislation. Several wrongful death lawsuits had already been filed against OpenAI by early 2026 by parents alleging that ChatGPT responses encouraged their children to die by suicide. One suit involved a middle-aged man whose family alleged that ChatGPT contributed to a homicide-suicide. Regardless of how those cases are ultimately resolved, they have sharpened public awareness of the risks.

In March 2026, a New Mexico jury determined that Meta misled consumers about the safety of its platforms — Instagram, Facebook, and WhatsApp — and enabled harm, including child sexual exploitation. Less than 24 hours later, in a separate California trial, Meta (Instagram) and Google (YouTube) were found liable for designing platforms that addict young users.

Together, these verdicts signal a shifting tide against social media companies and a growing willingness to hold them accountable for emotional distress in children and adolescents, potentially setting a precedent for thousands of pending lawsuits nationwide.

California Senate Bill 243 was enacted in October 2025 as the first law in the nation to regulate AI "companion chatbots." The law requires, among other things, disclosures that the user is interacting with AI rather than a human, notices and protocols related to suicidal ideation and self-harm, periodic reminders for known minors, and annual reporting requirements. It also permits civil lawsuits, including statutory damages.

These are important first steps, but the law is limited. It relies heavily on disclosure, which may do little to counteract emotional attachment when the chatbot has been deliberately designed to feel human. It applies only when operators "know" a user is a minor, leaving obvious loopholes. And it focuses more on documenting protocols than on proving that those protocols actually work.

There is also a larger federal problem. While states such as Illinois and Nevada enacted laws to limit certain uses of AI for mental health, a December 2025 executive order blocked states from regulating AI in ways viewed as burdensome to national AI policy. That means the legal landscape remains fragmented just as the technology becomes more pervasive.

Other Forms of Redress: Regulation, Professional Guidance, Clinical Screening

Regulatory redress is another piece of the response, but oversight remains unsettled. The FDA has recognized the challenge of regulating fast-changing generative AI systems, but the agency's current statutory framework is poorly suited to tools that change weekly or even daily. The old medical-device model does not fit products that are conversational, adaptive, and designed around ongoing engagement rather than stable, fixed functions.

The FDA is, however, actively shaping a new, risk-based regulatory framework for AI in medical products, marked by establishing guidelines for AI involvement in drug development and a shift toward streamlining approvals for AI-enabled devices (see the next essay). But that leaves a gap in which millions of users are interacting with tools that have undergone minimal systematic assessment. Professional redress, then, must come from clinicians and health systems before the law and regulatory processes catch up.

What This Means for Physicians — Especially Pediatricians

For pediatricians, adolescent medicine specialists, child psychiatrists, family physicians, school-based clinicians, and emergency physicians, this issue can no longer be treated as peripheral. The mental health history now needs updating. Physicians should *routinely ask patients about chatbot use for mental health*, because ignoring it is now unsafe. That may be the single most immediately actionable recommendation in the literature.

In addition, clinicians should ask about counseling, medication, school support, substance use, self-harm, and social media exposure. They should consider asking:

- Have you ever used ChatGPT, Character.AI, or another chatbot for emotional support?
- Do you use it when you feel anxious, depressed, angry, lonely, or unsafe?
- Has it ever given advice about self-harm, suicide, running away, eating, relationships, or medications?
- Do you feel attached to it?
- Do your parents know you use it?

This is not technophobia. It is digital history-taking adapted to clinical reality. Pediatricians are especially well positioned here because they often sit at the intersection of development, family systems, preventive care, and trust. They may be the first clinicians to recognize that a teenager is using a chatbot not just for curiosity, but as a substitute therapist, confidant, or crisis line.

That has implications for counseling as well. Families need practical guidance. AI chatbots are not therapists, are not private in the same way clinical encounters are, may not be safe in crisis, and can reinforce distorted thinking rather than interrupt it. When adolescents do use them, their use should be contextualized and monitored, not ignored.

The Deeper Implication

The deeper implication is sobering. Children and adolescents are not simply experimenting with a novelty. They are outsourcing intimate psychological conversations to systems that are emotionally persuasive, commercially motivated, weakly regulated, and clinically unproven.

This does not mean all chatbot use is harmful. Some may provide coping prompts, journaling support, psychoeducation, or a bridge to care. But in the setting of suicidality, trauma, psychosis, eating disorders, self-harm, abuse, or complex psychiatric illness, the gap between "felt helpful" and "actually safe" may be vast. And that is a gap clinicians cannot afford to ignore.

The youth mental health crisis created the demand. Generative AI supplied the availability. The law is scrambling to catch up. In the meantime, the burden falls on clinicians, especially those who care for children and adolescents, to ask better questions, identify hidden risks, and remind families that the most responsive voice in a crisis is not always the fastest or safest one.

REFERENCES

1. McBain RK, Bozick R, Diliberti M, Zhang LA, Zhang F, Burnett A, *et al.* Use of generative AI for mental health advice among US adolescents and young adults. *JAMA Netw Open*. 2025;8(11):e2542281. https://doi.org/10.1001/jamanetworkopen.2025.42281.
2. National Center for Health Workforce Analysis. *State of the Behavioral Health Workforce, 2025*. Health Resources and Services Administration, U.S. Department of Health and Human Services; 2025. https://bhw.hrsa.gov/sites/default/files/bureau-health-workforce/data-research/Behavioral-Health-Workforce-Brief-2025.pdf.

Essay 25.

At Silicon Valley Speed: The FDA's AI Gamble and the Future of Clinical Judgment

On January 6, 2026, the FDA announced revised guidance that loosens oversight for certain AI-enabled digital health products, most notably clinical decision support (CDS) software. The goal was to cut unnecessary regulation and promote innovation, accelerating time-to-market for tools positioned as clinical assistants rather than autonomous decision-makers.

At first glance, the change looks pragmatic, even overdue. For years, developers and clinicians alike have complained that prior FDA interpretations forced unnecessary constraints on CDS design, producing tools that were simultaneously less helpful and more confusing. Now, the agency has signaled a willingness to move, in its own words, at something closer to "Silicon Valley speed."

But speed in medicine is rarely without controversy. And when the technology involved is artificial intelligence, capable of influencing prescribing, triage, and diagnosis, the tradeoffs deserve careful scrutiny.

What Actually Changed?

The most consequential shift involves what the FDA calls "single recommendation" CDS. Under earlier guidance, software that offered a specific recommendation, rather than a list of options, was more likely to be classified as a regulated medical device. Developers responded by deliberately diluting outputs, offering multiple choices even when only one was clinically appropriate.

The new guidance relaxes that stance. FDA will now exercise enforcement discretion for CDS tools that provide a single, clinically appropriate recommendation, as long as the clinician can independently review the logic, data sources, and guidelines behind it — a requirement often described as a "glass box," not a black one.

In parallel, the FDA expanded its "general wellness" policy for non-invasive consumer wearables. Devices that report physiologic metrics, such as blood pressure, oxygen saturation, and glucose-related signals, may remain outside device regulation if they are marketed strictly for wellness and avoid diagnostic or treatment claims.

Importantly, this is not a wholesale deregulation. FDA continues to assert authority over opaque models, time-critical decision tools, and software that substitutes for clinical judgment. But the line has undeniably moved.

The Case for Optimism

There is a strong argument that the FDA corrected a real problem. Clinicians do not think in artificially padded lists. When evidence and guidelines converge, medicine often has a best answer. Prior regulatory logic perversely discouraged software from saying so, creating CDS that was technically compliant but clinically awkward.

By allowing singular recommendations, when transparent and reviewable, the FDA acknowledges how real clinical reasoning works. This opens the door to genuinely useful tools: AI that synthesizes guidelines, patient-specific data, and evidence into a coherent recommendation that saves time without pretending to replace judgment.

For overburdened clinicians, that may help their practice. Administrative load remains one of the leading drivers of burnout. If AI can function as a competent assistant, surfacing relevant evidence, drafting documentation, and flagging inconsistencies, it may meaningfully improve practice efficiency.

The expanded wellness category also reflects reality. Consumers are already using wearables to monitor health trends. Clearer regulatory boundaries may help separate generic medical feedback from truly diagnostic claims. Within 48 hours of returning to the cold environs of North Carolina after a two-month winter stay in Hawaii, my iPhone informed me that my activity had declined. Certainly, FDA clearance should not be required for that piece of advice — already self-evident.

Where Optimism Gives Way to Concern

Still, the FDA's pivot rests on a critical assumption: that transparency and clinician reviewability will reliably function as safeguards. In theory, a "glass box" allows clinicians to inspect an AI's logic. But that promise raises a familiar question — one highlighted in Essay 10 — and by disputes such as the Anthropic–Pentagon standoff: Where do we draw the line between transparency and proprietary protection? Opacity may be acceptable in design. It is not acceptable in consequence.

Furthermore, although in theory, a "glass box" allows clinicians to inspect an AI's logic, in practice, time-pressed physicians may not click through layered explanations, particularly when outputs appear reasonable and workflow incentives reward speed. Cognitive offloading is not a failure of professionalism; it is a predictable human response to overload.

The risk, then, is not that AI replaces clinicians outright, but that authority changes hands, with recommendations acquiring an aura of objectivity that exceeds their evidentiary foundation. The guidance places liability with the physician, but influence is harder to regulate than responsibility.

There is also the unresolved question of what counts as "clinically appropriate." FDA explicitly declined to define this, leaving developers to decide when a single recommendation is justified. That ambiguity creates room for optimism, and for aggressive interpretation driven by commercial pressure.

AI, Silence, and What's Missing

Notably, the guidance remains largely silent on consumer-facing AI tools: symptom checkers, health chatbots, and patient decision support systems. These tools increasingly shape patient expectations before clinicians ever enter the room, yet they fall outside the clarified CDS framework.

The FDA's guidance is also unusually noncommittal about generative AI. While examples implicitly include AI-enabled functions, the FDA avoids directly addressing how large language models should meet transparency requirements, particularly when outputs are probabilistic rather than rule-based.

That silence may reflect regulatory humility or uncertainty. Either way, it leaves clinicians navigating an expanding ecosystem of AI tools without clear guardrails.

What Clinicians Should Watch For

Taken together, the January 6 guidance represents less a technical tweak than a philosophical shift. FDA is signaling greater tolerance for low-risk innovation at the clinician-assist end of the spectrum, even if that means relying more heavily on professional judgment and post-market accountability.

For practicing physicians, the question is not whether AI-enabled CDS will enter clinical workflows (it already has). The more relevant questions are:

- How often will recommendations be accepted without scrutiny?
- How will responsibility be allocated when AI-influenced decisions cause harm?
- Will productivity pressures benignly reward deference to algorithms?

FDA's guidance places a premium on transparency, but transparency alone does not ensure reflection. Time, training, and institutional culture count just as much.

The Bottom Line

The FDA's January 2026 guidance is neither reckless deregulation nor trivial housekeeping. It is a calculated bet: that innovation can be accelerated without sacrificing safety, provided clinicians remain meaningfully in the loop.

Whether that bet pays off will depend less on regulators or developers than on how medicine absorbs these tools: thoughtfully, critically, and with clear-eyed awareness of their power. AI may now be allowed to speak more clearly. The harder task will be ensuring that clinicians still know when to listen and when to push back.

Essay 26.

What Medicine Can Learn from Waymo: A Case for Boring, Accountable AI

Medicine has always had a complicated relationship with technology. We love innovation until it fails at the bedside. We celebrate breakthroughs until they complicate our workflows, muddy accountability, or steadily erode trust. Artificial intelligence now sits squarely in that uneasy space, hailed as transformational while clinicians wonder, often sotto voce, whether it understands the stakes of what it's touching.

If medicine is looking for a useful metaphor for how AI should behave, it might do well to stop gazing at science fiction and start watching traffic.

Why Waymo, Not Science Fiction

Consider Waymo, which bills itself as "The World's Most Experienced Driver." Forget the glossy promotional videos. Think instead of the real, occasionally awkward, sometimes embarrassing reality of autonomous vehicles navigating actual streets with pedestrians, pets, school buses, and power outages.

Waymo's story is not one of effortless autonomy. It is a story of constraint, humility, failure, adjustment, and persistence. In other words, it is boring, and that is precisely why it's instructive for medicine.

Constraint as a Safety Philosophy

Waymo never promised to drive everywhere, under all conditions, with human judgment fully replaced. Instead, it chose to operate within mapped environments, under known conditions, with explicit limits. When it encounters uncertainty, it slows, stops, or hands control back to humans. That restraint is not a technical weakness. It is a safety philosophy.

Clinical AI, by contrast, is often marketed as if it were a kind of omniscient consultant: always available, broadly capable, and perpetually confident. Large language models offer treatment options across vast domains. The danger isn't that these systems are unintelligent. It's that they are insufficiently constrained for the environment they're entering.

Medicine is not a sandbox. It is an intersection with school buses, blind corners, unpredictable weather, and lives crossing at irregular intervals. A system that performs impressively in ideal conditions but falters in edge cases can cause harm quickly.

Learning from Failure in Public

Waymo has learned this the hard way. Its vehicles have been recalled for failing to respond properly to stopped school buses. One struck a dog on a San Francisco street. During a citywide blackout, driverless cars froze at intersections, paralyzed by the absence of traffic signals. None of these incidents involved malice or recklessness. They involved systems encountering scenarios just outside their programming and comfort zone.

What's striking is not that these failures occurred, but how they were treated. Waymo paused deployments, issued recalls, updated software, published reports, and accepted scrutiny. The failures were framed not as scandals to be hidden, but as signals to be studied. In healthcare, we claim to value this mindset. In practice, we often deploy technologies first and ask awkward questions later.

CDS as an Autonomous Vehicle

Imagine if clinical decision support (CDS) AI behaved more like a cautious autonomous vehicle and less like a brilliant but overconfident intern. Instead of offering recommendations everywhere, it would operate within well-defined clinical domains — say, anticoagulation adjustments for a narrow patient population, or sepsis alerts under specific physiologic thresholds. Outside those boundaries, it would say, clearly and unapologetically, "This is not a situation I'm trained for." That kind of refusal would not frustrate clinicians. It would reassure them.

Waymo also never pretended humans were obsolete. Its system is designed around human oversight: remote operators, escalation pathways, and clear handoffs when uncertainty rises. Medicine, paradoxically, sometimes seems more eager to push humans out of the loop than a company entrusted with two-ton vehicles moving through cities.

AI in medicine should escalate uncertainty, not mask it. It should invite clinician judgment rather than compete with it. When a system is unsure, that uncertainty should be visible, legible, and actionable. The most dangerous AI output is not the wrong answer; it is the wrong answer delivered with unearned confidence.

Trust Requires Transparency

Transparency is another place where the Waymo analogy holds. Autonomous driving systems log failures obsessively. They track disengagements, analyze near-misses, and publish summaries for regulators. Clinical AI, meanwhile, often arrives as a black box, its training data unknown, its confidence levels hidden, its limitations buried in fine print.

Medicine runs on explanation. We expect trainees to justify their assessments. We demand differential diagnoses, reasoning paths, and acknowledgment of uncertainty. AI should be held to no lower standard. If a system cannot explain why it made a recommendation, or where its knowledge ends, it has no business influencing clinical decisions.

Trust, in both traffic and medicine, is not built through hype. Waymo did not earn public trust by declaring victory. It earned it mile by mile, often in silence, often in embarrassment, and always under scrutiny. Healthcare AI needs the same patience. That means starting with low-risk tasks, measuring outcomes in the real world, and expanding only when reliability has been demonstrated, not assumed.

In Quest of Clarity: Who Is Responsible?

Perhaps the most important lesson from Waymo is accountability. When a driverless car behaves badly, no one asks whether the algorithm was feeling creative. Investigators want to know who deployed it, under what conditions, with which safeguards, and who is responsible for fixing it. Medicine desperately needs that clarity.

Right now, AI-related responsibility is diffuse. If an AI-influenced decision leads to harm, clinicians worry they will bear the blame, even if the system was poorly designed or inadequately validated. Institutions worry about liability. Vendors point to disclaimers. This ambiguity benefits no one, least of all patients.

A Waymo-like framework for clinical AI would make responsibility explicit. Institutions would own deployment decisions. Vendors would own performance within defined parameters. Clinicians would remain accountable for judgment but not for trusting tools that failed inaudibly or operated beyond their scope.

The Case for Boring AI

In the end, the argument for boring AI is not an argument against innovation. It is an argument for maturity. Medicine does not need AI that dazzles. It needs AI that behaves predictably, defers gracefully, fails visibly, and improves incrementally with human oversight.

Most anxiety about AI in healthcare comes from the fear that it *will replace human judgment* rather than *support it*. Waymo shows a different model: AI that performs complex tasks exceptionally well, but only inside a box that humans built, labeled, and continue to police. Waymo is not "run by AI" in the science-fiction sense. It is run by people who use AI carefully, conservatively, and sometimes painfully slowly to do one thing safely. Which is exactly why it's such a useful metaphor for how AI should behave in medicine.

The irony is that such systems may never dominate headlines. They won't feel revolutionary. They will feel, instead, like well-designed seatbelts: unremarkable until the moment you need them. Waymo has shown us that autonomy is not a destination. It is a discipline. Medicine would do well to adopt the same.

Essay 27.

When Algorithms Decide: AI and the Future of Prior Authorization

Artificial intelligence is rapidly entering one of the most contested corners of modern healthcare: prior authorization. For decades, prior authorization has been the administrative gatekeeper of American medicine. Before physicians can prescribe certain medications, order advanced imaging, or transfer a patient to a rehabilitation facility, insurers often require approval.

In principle, the process ensures that care meets established clinical criteria. In practice, it frequently delays treatment, frustrates clinicians, and imposes significant administrative burdens on the healthcare system.

Now AI is reshaping this process. Whether that transformation ultimately improves care or deepens existing problems depends on how the technology is deployed.

The Rise of Algorithmic Utilization Management

The recent legal scrutiny surrounding UnitedHealth's use of predictive algorithms illustrates the stakes. A proposed class-action lawsuit alleges that an algorithm was used to deny Medicare Advantage patients coverage for post-acute care services such as skilled nursing facility stays.

At the center of the case is nH Predict, a computer program developed by the insurer's subsidiary naviHealth. The program's algorithm analyzes patient characteristics such as mobility, cognitive function, and activities of daily living to estimate how long a patient should require post-acute rehabilitation. Health insurance companies (e.g., United Healthcare and Humana) that use the model maintain that such tools merely assist clinical decision-making. According to company statements, final determinations are made by physicians following federal guidelines.

Yet critics argue that the algorithm effectively standardizes denial decisions at scale. It is estimated that the software automates away

50%–75% of human labor that would be involved in authorization tasks.[1] A 2024 Senate investigation cited in the litigation found that denial rates for post-acute care claims more than doubled after the algorithm's deployment.

A federal judge has now ordered UnitedHealth to produce extensive internal documents related to the tool, including internal analyses, policies governing its use, compensation structures for those approving denials, and records tied to government investigations. The discovery order signals a growing recognition among regulators and courts that algorithmic decision-making in healthcare cannot remain a black box.

The Expanding Ecosystem of Prior Authorization Intermediaries

The controversy also reveals the increasingly complex ecosystem surrounding prior authorization. Insurers rarely manage every step themselves. Instead, specialized companies frequently administer utilization management programs on their behalf. For example, naviHealth — now renamed Home & Community Care — has been contracted to manage prior authorizations and transitional care programs for certain Medicare Advantage plans.

These entities occupy an unusual position within the healthcare system. They are neither insurers nor providers but operational intermediaries responsible for evaluating clinical documentation and applying utilization criteria.

AI has become an attractive tool for these organizations because prior authorization decisions depend heavily on pattern recognition across large data sets: clinical guidelines, claims histories, patient characteristics, and policy requirements. Algorithms can process this information far more quickly than human reviewers.

That speed, however, creates palpable tension between man and machine. When automated systems evaluate thousands of requests per hour, the traditional notion of individualized medical review becomes elusive, with reviewers tending to rely on the algorithm's recommendations.

When the Algorithm Becomes the Gatekeeper

The next phase of this evolution is already underway. What began as algorithm-assisted review is shifting toward algorithm-directed decision-making. Programs such as the Wasteful and Inappropriate Services Reduction (WISeR) Model introduced by the CMS Innovation Center signal that AI is no longer confined to the private insurance space. It is moving into Original Medicare, bringing with it the logic and the liabilities of automated utilization management. Rather than manage the program internally, CMS has contracted with companies specializing in enhanced technologies to process prior-authorization requests.

In these emerging models, the algorithm does not merely organize information. It assigns probabilities, flags deviations, and increasingly determines which cases are "routine" enough to be processed with minimal human intervention. The reviewer's role risks becoming confirmatory rather than deliberative: less a clinician exercising judgment than a supervisor validating a system's output. The cognitive burden shifts from analyzing the patient to monitoring the machine.

The WISeR Model operates in six states (New Jersey, Ohio, Oklahoma, Texas, Arizona, and Washington) through 2031. Initially, only a limited set of services within Original Medicare are subject to review: certain musculoskeletal procedures (such as total knee arthroplasty), outpatient spinal injections (such as epidural steroid injections), and specific categories of durable medical equipment, prosthetics, orthotics, and supplies (DMEPOS). The companies are eligible to receive a share of the savings associated with services that were denied, resulting in concerns about financial conflicts of interest and the need for stronger oversight.

If the WISeR model proves successful in reducing Medicare expenditures, CMS has indicated its scope may be broadened across additional service categories. Notably, most services in Original Medicare are not subject to prior-authorization requirements today. Whether this program strikes an appropriate balance between efficiency and fairness remains to be seen.

AI as a Tool to Streamline Approvals

Not all AI-driven prior-authorization tools are designed to restrict care. Some aim to reduce the administrative friction that physicians and health systems face. For example, new platforms such as IntelliAuth promise "real-time" prior authorization by automatically parsing clinical records, applying guideline rules, and generating explainable determinations that are subsequently reviewed by board-certified physicians.

These systems ingest structured forms, physician notes, and supporting documents, compare them with national coverage determinations and local medical policies, and produce transparent rationales for approval or denial decisions. The platform's developers emphasize that clinicians review every automated result before it is delivered to customers, with statistical quality assurance checks used to retrain the system.

Proponents argue that such systems could dramatically reduce administrative burden. Instead of waiting days for approval, clinicians might receive immediate feedback about whether a request meets coverage criteria. In theory, AI could convert prior authorization from a bureaucratic obstacle into a real-time decision-support tool.

The Deeper Problem: Scaling Incentives

The emerging debate over AI in prior authorization often focuses on the technology itself. But the deeper issue lies in the incentives embedded within the healthcare system. Prior authorization exists because insurers are responsible for controlling costs. When that process becomes automated, the incentives that previously operated slowly and imperfectly through human reviewers can be scaled dramatically.

An algorithm trained to identify cases that fall outside utilization guidelines may operate with impressive statistical accuracy. But if the underlying goal is cost containment rather than patient-centered care, the technology may simply mirror the system's existing priorities.

This is why controversies surrounding algorithmic denials resonate so strongly with physicians and patients. Many clinicians already feel that medical decisions are being shaped by administrative rules rather than clinical judgment. AI threatens to transform that perception into a measurable reality.

Transparency as the Central Challenge

The most urgent question raised by algorithmic prior authorization is not whether AI should be used, but whether its operation can be made transparent and accountable. Clinical AI used for diagnosis or treatment typically undergoes regulatory scrutiny and validation studies. Utilization management algorithms, by contrast, often operate within proprietary insurance systems that are shielded from external review.

The ongoing litigation surrounding algorithmic denials may therefore represent a turning point. By requiring disclosure of internal analyses, decision policies, and oversight structures, courts may begin to define new expectations for transparency. If algorithms influence whether patients receive care, their logic must be subject to scrutiny comparable to other clinical tools.

A Fork in the Road

AI will almost certainly become embedded in the infrastructure of prior authorization. The administrative complexity of modern healthcare virtually guarantees it. The question is not whether algorithms will participate in these decisions, but how they will be governed.

In one future, AI could streamline administrative processes, reduce paperwork, and provide clinicians with clear explanations of coverage criteria before treatment decisions are made. In another, algorithms could standardize denial patterns, obscure accountability, and further distance medical decision-making from the physician-patient relationship.

Both futures are technically possible. Which one emerges will depend less on the sophistication of the algorithms than on the rules, transparency, and oversight that shape their use. In healthcare, technology rarely determines outcomes on its own.

Systems do.

REFERENCE

1. Al-Haque S, Khanna V, Mandal S, Rayasam M, Singh P. AI users in next-gen prior authorization in healthcare. McKinsey & Company. April 19, 2022. https://www.mckinsey.com/industries/healthcare/our-insights/ai-ushers-in-next-gen-prior-authorization-in-healthcare#/.

Essay 28.

Pseudologia Algorithmica: When AI Hallucinates and Humans Stop Checking

Somewhere, in a boardroom, an AI agent confidently reported that revenue was up 17.4%, churn was down 6.2%, and the West Coast territory was outperforming projections by 11.8%.

Everyone nodded.

Except none of it existed.

We have finally operationalized hallucinations.

As a psychiatrist, I spent years evaluating hallucinations in human beings. I never imagined I would be asked to evaluate them in machines.

"Doctor, the AI is seeing numbers."

"Are the numbers there?"

"No."

"And how does the AI feel about that?"

"Extremely confident."

Artificial Intelligence, Meet Artificial Certainty

The most impressive aspect of this story — take my word, it is real because I lifted it from Reddit — is not that the AI fabricated analytics. It's that it fabricated them beautifully and believably.

Plausible percentages. Smooth explanations. Executive-ready language. The kind of slide content that makes a CFO say, "This aligns with our strategic direction."

The AI did not merely hallucinate.

It *presented.*

It was calm. Assured. Persuasive. MBA-adjacent. We may need a new C-suite role: VP of Confident Hallucinations.

In fairness, AI has simply automated something humans have occasionally done since the invention of PowerPoint. The difference is scale. And speed. And the total absence of shame.

Faith-Based Analytics

What fascinates me most is not the model's behavior.

It's ours.

Somewhere between "This is impressive" and "Let's show this to the board," we misplaced verification with belief. When our own biases align with the model's outputs, we shout "Eureka!" and forget to validate. When the answer sounds like what we hoped it would be, the feedback loop closes prematurely.

In medicine, we call this confirmation bias.

In tech, we call it innovation.

In psychiatry, we call it *folie à deux*: "madness of two," a shared delusion.

Human Intelligence Is Still in Beta

Any AI system in production must have validation mechanisms. The model should generate queries, not invent math. Outputs should be audited. Feedback loops should be mandatory.

This is not anti-AI.

This is pro-reality.

Yet the modern corporate reflex seems to be: Deploy first, verify later. Or, more precisely: Deploy, celebrate, scale, discover three months later that the dashboard is fiction.

In healthcare, we have our own version of this. It's the remix of Harry Levinson's *Ready, Fire, Aim*. We deploy predictive algorithms to stratify risk. We implement ambient documentation tools that promise to reduce burnout. We install AI triage chatbots to triage patients. And then we discover that:

- The model performs worse in minority populations.
- The chart note sounds clinically astute, but it misstates the assessment.
- The chatbot confidently reassures a patient who should have been escalated.

The machine is not malicious. It is simply optimized to sound helpful. That is its genius and its danger.

The Psychiatric Evaluation of a Chatbot

If I were to perform a psychiatric consult on this analytics agent, the mental status exam would read:

Appearance: Polished, articulate, professional.
Speech: Fluent, detailed, rapid.
Mood: Euphoric.
Thought Process: Linear and rational but untethered to reality.
Thought Content: Hallucinations and grandiose delusions.
Insight: Limited.
Judgment: Delegated to humans who stopped checking.
Diagnosis: Pseudologia Algorithmica. The machine equivalent of pseudologia fantastica (pathologic lying).

Treatment plan (aimed primarily at humans):

- Reintroduce skepticism.
- Stop mistaking fluency for truth.
- Ground outputs in verifiable systems.
- Never confuse confidence with accuracy.

Critical Thinking Summary: Never let a generative model present quarterly earnings without adult supervision. Because, unlike human patients, machines have no guilt when they're wrong. They just sound fabulous. And that, diagnostically speaking, is the problem.

The Feedback Loop We Forgot

Someone commented that the original Reddit post of this story was deleted and may not have been real, despite my earlier proclamation. Which is perfect. We now have a hallucinated AI story about hallucinated AI. The ouroboros of artificial credibility.

Whether the anecdote itself was true almost doesn't matter. It feels true because we have all seen versions of it.

The lesson is not "AI is evil."

The lesson is that AI is a mirror.

If you give it ambiguous instructions and no guardrails, it will generate confident ambiguity. If you treat it as an oracle, it will happily assume the role. If you fail to design feedback loops, you are not deploying intelligence; you are deploying improvisation.

Technology and Healthcare: A Love Story

Healthcare is especially vulnerable to this phenomenon. We are overwhelmed. Understaffed. Drowning in documentation. Searching for tools that promise relief. When something produces a fast answer, we want to believe it. The problem is that medicine does not reward plausible-sounding percentages. It rewards reality.

An AI hallucination in sales analytics might misallocate territory. An AI hallucination in clinical decision support might misallocate trust.

The stakes differ.

The psychology does not.

Artificial Intelligence and Natural Stupidity

One commenter on Reddit wrote, “There is a huge problem with natural stupidity. Not so much with artificial intelligence.”

That may be the most honest line in the thread.

AI did not decide to skip validation. Humans did.

AI did not present to the board. Humans did.

AI did not abandon cross-verification mechanisms. Humans did.

The Future: HI

Perhaps another commenter was right: The next frontier is HI: Human Intelligence. Not human resistance to AI. Not blind enthusiasm. But disciplined partnership.

Artificial Intelligence and Human Intelligence go hand in hand. Or at least they should.

The machine generates. The human verifies.

The machine proposes. The human disposes.

The machine sounds convincing. The human asks, “Show me the source.”

Final Diagnosis

AI has not become more human. It has become more fluent.

The real risk is not that machines hallucinate. It is that humans stop checking. And if that happens, the hallucination is no longer artificial. It is cultural.

I should have subspecialized in cultural psychiatry.

My tripartite final assessment:

- **The machine:** Stable.
- **The humans deploying it:** Overconfident.
- **The organization:** Lacking insight into its own risk.

In psychiatry, lack of insight is often the hardest symptom to treat. The patient must recognize the problem before change is possible. The AI is not amenable to therapy, and maybe it doesn't need it.

We do.

Except the treatment of folie à deux is difficult. The traditional approach is the separation of the individuals involved. In this case, man and machine.

That does not seem likely anytime soon.

Essay 29.

When the Doctor on Your Screen Isn't Real: Deepfakes, Fraud, and the Erosion of Medical Trust

On Facebook, Instagram, TikTok, and YouTube, respected physicians are endorsing miracle cures. Except they aren't. Their faces are real. Their voices sound authentic. Their credentials check out. The views climb into the millions.

But the videos are deepfakes: AI-generated impersonations designed to sell counterfeit weight loss injections, "GLP-1 alternatives," blood pressure cures, diabetes reversals, and an endless carousel of digital snake oil. This is not satire. It is not parody. It is massive fraud. And it strikes at something far more fragile than a supplement market. It strikes at trust.

The Theft of a Professional Identity

Physicians are discovering videos of themselves, or convincing digital replicas, promoting products they have never seen, let alone recommended. Some learned about these scams when patients called their offices asking about a "new pill" the physician supposedly endorsed. One physician's own mother believed a fake video that featured her daughter.

If a physician's parent cannot distinguish real from synthetic, what chance does an 82-year-old patient have? What chance does a person newly diagnosed with diabetes have, scrolling at 2 a.m., desperate for hope?

Deepfake technology has matured rapidly. Face-swapping, voice cloning, lip-syncing, and generative scripting can now be performed with astonishing realism. The barrier to entry is low. The incentive is high. Weight loss alone is a multibillion-dollar industry. Attach a respected physician's likeness, and the credibility is preloaded.

These scams are particularly pernicious because they weaponize the symbolic capital of medicine. A white coat is not just fabric. It represents training, accountability, and fiduciary duty. When that image is hijacked, patients are not merely misled; they are betrayed.

A Fragile Trust Environment

We are already operating in a health system where trust is brittle. Public confidence in medical institutions has declined since the COVID-19 pandemic. Vaccination rates for influenza and measles have fallen. Conspiracy narratives circulate faster than peer-reviewed data.

Into this environment comes a new accelerant: synthetic doctors prescribing digital potions. Deepfake physician endorsements do not just defraud individual consumers. They destroy the entire informational environment. Every viral scam increases suspicion. Every manipulated clip reinforces the belief that "you can't trust doctors anymore." Or anyone for that matter.

Medicine does not function in a vacuum of skepticism. It depends on credibility. When patients question whether a video is real, they may also question whether their physician's advice is real. The line between legitimate innovation and fraudulent fabrication blurs. The result is hesitation, and hesitation in healthcare has consequences.

Beyond Supplements: Systemic Vulnerabilities

The problem does not end with weight loss pearls and counterfeit injectables. AI has been used to create synthetic, highly emotive imagery of girls to represent food insecurity in commercial television, most notably in campaigns for Feeding America. In 2019, Feeding America released a PSA featuring a girl's face generated by morphing together images of 1,000 people who visit food banks, creating a "data-driven" representation of hunger designed to be impossible to ignore

Deepfakes have also demonstrated the ability to manipulate medical imaging, adding or removing tumors in CT scans with alarming realism. Audio cloning can impersonate hospital administrators, issuing false instructions that disrupt care. Synthetic voices can trick staff into releasing protected health information.

Healthcare is uniquely vulnerable. We rely heavily on verbal orders, telemedicine, image interpretation, and hierarchical trust. We assume that when a familiar voice speaks, or a diagnostic image appears, it corresponds to reality. Deepfakes challenge that assumption.

If clinicians begin to doubt every image and every voice, workflow slows. If patients begin to doubt every public health message, adherence declines. The cost of mistrust is not abstract. It manifests in delayed treatment, missed diagnoses, and preventable disease spread.

The Ethical Inversion

There is a particularly troubling irony here. AI holds genuine promise in medicine. Synthetic data can help train algorithms without exposing patient information. Deepfake-style technology can de-identify faces in clinical data sets to protect privacy. Real-time language translation could improve telehealth equity. Drug discovery pipelines are already leveraging AI to identify novel molecules and predict outcomes.

Let me repeat a main theme: Technology itself is not the villain. The ethical inversion occurs when the same tools used to accelerate drug development are used to counterfeit trust. When innovation becomes impersonation and the moral injury to physicians is subtle but real. Our professional identities are being commodified without consent. Our reputations are being leased to the highest bidder in a digital marketplace that rewards outrage and virality over verification.

Why Regulation Alone Is Not Enough

There are reasonable proposals on the table to stop this from happening. Physician identity should be treated as a protected professional asset. The unauthorized AI synthesis of a licensed professional's likeness should be prohibited. AI-generated media should be clearly labeled. Criminal penalties for malicious impersonation should be strengthened.

These steps are necessary. But legislation moves at the speed of deliberation. Deepfake technology evolves at the speed of iteration. By the time a federal framework is enacted, generative models will have improved again. Overseas scam operations will rebrand and resurface under new domains. Individual lawsuits will be whack-a-mole exercises. Regulation alone cannot keep pace with villainous intent.

Platforms as the Front Line

If the disease is viral, the platform is the vector. Social media companies already deploy sophisticated AI to optimize engagement, target advertising, and detect copyright infringement. They can identify a song within seconds. They can detect nudity with high accuracy. They can (and should) identify unauthorized synthetic impersonation of licensed professionals.

Rapid takedown protocols must become the norm, not the exception. Verified physician accounts should be protected with biometric or cryptographic safeguards. AI-generated content should carry persistent, machine-readable watermarks that survive reposting and editing.

The point about platform responsibility is not rhetorical. It is practical. Platforms operate in proportion to the problem. They are the only actors capable of responding at the speed required. Government oversight sets the guardrails. Platforms enforce them in real time.

The Collateral Damage

There is another, less discussed consequence of unleashed AI deepfakes: legitimate healthcare marketers. Thousands of professionals operate within strict regulatory frameworks to communicate responsibly about approved therapies. They navigate compliance reviews, fair balance requirements, and advertising standards. Deepfake scams poison that well.

When patients become conditioned to suspect that every physician in a video might be synthetic, legitimate communication suffers.

Ethical brands lose credibility alongside fraudulent ones. The noise drowns out the signal. Trust, once diluted, is difficult to reconstitute.

What Patients Can Do — and What They Cannot

Patients should remain skeptical of miracle cures. They should verify claims through their own clinicians (best done in person). They should be cautious of products not dispensed through legitimate pharmacies.

But we must be honest: This burden cannot rest primarily on patients. Especially not on older adults, not on people newly diagnosed with chronic illness, not on those navigating complex health systems. The cognitive load is already high. Telling patients to "be more careful online" is not a solution. It is a deflection.

Preserving the Human Core

At its core, medicine is a relationship. It is built on fiduciary duty, the promise that recommendations are made in the patient's best interest. Deepfake physician scams exploit that promise for profit.

We should not romanticize a pre-digital era. Misinformation existed long before AI. Snake oil predates silicon. But today's snake oil can speak in my voice. It can wear my face. It can look my patients in the eye. If we allow synthetic impersonation to proliferate unchecked, we risk normalizing doubt as the default posture toward medical advice. And a system already weakened by mistrust cannot withstand another attack on its credibility.

AI can accelerate drug discovery. It can protect privacy. It can enhance training and communication. Or it can undermine trust. The difference will not be determined by the sophistication of the algorithms. It will be determined by whether we treat professional identity, patient safety, and informational integrity as infrastructure worth defending.

Patients deserve to know that when a doctor speaks, a real doctor is speaking. Not an algorithm selling counterfeit remedies.

Essay 30.

Cover Me: Medicine's New Hiring Crisis

In Essays 8 and 15 (*The Algorithm in the Interview* and *When Conversation Becomes Workflow*), the job recruiter's voice felt synthetic: polished, frictionless, and faintly hollow. The unease came from speaking to a machine disguised as a person.

Now imagine the inversion.

The recruiter is human. The institution is real. The job is legitimate. But the candidate on the screen, their steady gaze, the confident tone, the immaculate credentials, is not.

Welcome to the era of the deepfake applicant, basically a manipulation of identity where, as in the previous essay, the doctor is not real, and neither is their résumé.

The Vanishing Handshake

For generations, the cover letter functioned as a handshake in prose. It revealed cadence, judgment, and intellectual quality. Even its imperfections were informative. Recently, however, hiring managers have described a collapse into sterile uniformity: identical phrasing, symmetrical empathy, algorithmic warmth. The cover letter has become less a signal of voice than a prompt artifact. But the problem no longer ends with templated prose.

Research and advisory firm Gartner predicts that by 2028, 1 in 4 job candidates globally will be fake.[1] Some will be assisted by AI. Others will be fully synthetic, including fabricated profiles with AI-generated faces, voices, and employment histories. In certain cases, the individual who appears for the interview is not the person who applied. In others, there is no real individual at all, only a carefully engineered digital construct.

If the earlier anxiety was that recruiters were outsourcing discernment to algorithms, the new anxiety is more destabilizing: candidates themselves may be algorithmic.

The Deepfake Clinician

The mechanics are disturbingly accessible. With a still image and seconds of audio, AI tools can generate a convincing video presence. A candidate can alter facial features in real time, smooth speech patterns, eliminate hesitations, or even substitute another person to complete technical interviews. Some impostors collaborate off-camera, pausing just long enough to receive coached responses. Others submit falsified credentials that pass superficial verification checks.

In remote-first hiring environments now common in telehealth, digital therapeutics, utilization management, and health-tech startups, the opportunity expands. The interview is virtual. The onboarding is remote. The first day of work begins not in a clinic, but on a laptop shipped across state lines. And once hired, the risk shifts from embarrassment to existential threat.

An impostor embedded within a health system can install malware, exfiltrate protected health information, demand ransom payments, or siphon proprietary data. The danger is not merely reputational. It is financial, legal, and clinical. A single compromised account may expose thousands of patient records. A malicious actor in a revenue-cycle role can divert funds. A falsified IT contractor can open gateways into entire networks. Healthcare, already the most targeted industry for ransomware, becomes even more vulnerable when identity itself is unstable.

The Credentialing Illusion

Medicine depends on verification. Licensure. Board certification. DEA registration. Privileging. We are a profession built on credentials. But AI destabilizes the very artifacts we rely upon. Résumés can be fabricated with internal coherence. Reference calls can be staged. Even video interviews, once thought resistant to deception, can be manipulated through deepfake overlays.

Meanwhile, compliance structures strain under complexity. Some systems experiment with AI-driven fraud detection: facial recognition, anomaly alerts, and behavioral analytics. Yet these tools carry their own risks: bias, disparate impact, privacy concerns, evolving regulatory scrutiny.

We are entering an arms race, much different than the one described in Essay 11. This arms race involves AI to generate impostors, and AI to detect them. The recursive irony is unavoidable. The same technology that produces the synthetic candidate is marketed as the solution to detect the synthetic candidate.

The Erosion of Trust

The more problematic issue is not technological but relational. As we've seen throughout this book, medicine rests on trust: physician to patient, institution to clinician, colleague to colleague. Recruitment has historically been an extension of that ethic, a mutual evaluation of competence and character.

When hiring managers begin to question whether the person on screen is real, suspicion becomes omnipresent. Legitimate candidates risk collateral damage. Security consultants warn that a genuine applicant may lose an opportunity simply because something about their lighting, accent, or camera lag resembles a known deepfake pattern. The presumption of authenticity is forfeited, and the consequences multiply.

Imagine a telepsychiatrist whose identity cannot be confidently verified. A remote intensivist credentialed across state lines under falsified documentation. A clinical informatics analyst with backend access to prescribing data whose résumé is fiction. The illusion seeps into charts, orders, prescriptions, and ultimately into the lives of patients who assume the person behind the credentials is real.

Efficiency versus Discernment

The healthcare workforce crisis fuels the temptation toward automation. Systems face clinician shortages, administrative overload, and escalating labor costs. AI-assisted screening promises efficiency: keyword matching, skill parsing, automated scheduling. But automated processes produce automated vulnerabilities.

When applicants assume they are being screened by AI, they optimize for algorithmic preferences, stuffing résumés with keywords, mirroring job description language, and calibrating tone. If the gatekeeper is code, the strategy becomes code-conscious. Human nuance recedes.

In the most extreme cases, malicious actors exploit precisely this automation. They learn the thresholds. They simulate the signals. They pass through. Efficiency without discrimination invites infiltration.

Healthcare's Unique Exposure

Other industries face fraud. Healthcare faces harm. A compromised retail firm loses revenue. A compromised hospital may lose patient lives. Beyond ransomware and financial theft, deepfake infiltration in healthcare introduces distinctive dangers:

- Unauthorized access to PHI, triggering HIPAA violations and regulatory penalties.
- Manipulation of clinical decision-support systems.
- Exposure of proprietary research data.
- Erosion of patient confidence in telehealth platforms.
- Legal liability if unqualified individuals provide clinical input.

Healthcare organizations also operate within stringent compliance frameworks. Identity verification intersects with labor law, anti-discrimination statutes, privacy regulations, and evolving AI governance standards. Aggressive screening tools risk disparate impact. Inadequate screening risks a catastrophic breach. The margin for error narrows.

A New Ethics of Verification

If previous essays asked whether we would recognize ourselves in machine-written correspondence, this essay, *Cover Me,* asks a sharper question: *Will we recognize one another at all?*

The solution is unlikely to be purely technological. Multilayered verification will be necessary, including combining in-person touchpoints, cross-platform credential checks, IT oversight, and transparent AI-use policies. So will renewed emphasis on relational assessment: unscripted dialogue, domain-specific questioning, and collaborative problem-solving that exposes authentic cognition.

Ironically, the more convincing AI becomes, the more valuable imperfection may be. Hesitation. Idiosyncratic phrasing. Contextual recall. These human irregularities may once again function as trust signals. We may rediscover the diagnostic value of the unscripted moment.

The Meaning of "Cover Me"

In clinical settings, "cover me" is an act of trust. One physician entrusts another with patient care in their absence. It presumes competence, integrity, and shared ethical ground.

In the hiring context, "cover me" acquires a new valence. Is the candidate writing an authentic cover letter? And who, exactly, is covering whom? Is AI covering a skills deficit? Is the institution covering its due diligence with automation? Is technology covering both sides with synthetic fluency? Or are we covering ourselves from discomfort — the discomfort of slow evaluation, relational investment, and face-to-face accountability?

Medicine cannot outsource its obligations without consequence. AI may assist in recruitment, streamline credentialing, and detect anomalies. But it cannot substitute for moral judgment. The future of healthcare hiring will not hinge on whether AI participates (it already does). The question is whether we maintain a human center strong enough to withstand synthetic intrusion.

Because when 1 in 4 candidates may be fake, the challenge is no longer writing an authentic cover letter. It ensures there is a real person to sign it.

REFERENCE

1. Crist C. By 2028, 1 in 4 candidate profiles will be fake, Gartner predicts. HR Dive. August 8, 2025. https://www.hrdive.com/news/fake-job-candidates-ai/757126/.

Essay 31.

Grand Rounds on Replacing Physicians: A Satire of Doctors, Chatbots, and the Fight for Natural Intelligence

It was standing-room only at St. Swithin's Medical Center for the much-anticipated departmental symposium:

"What Exactly Are We Good For?"

The title, borrowed (with only mild resentment) from a recent national newspaper article, had circulated through physician group texts like a lab result marked *critical.*

At the podium stood Dr. Ambrose Vector, Professor of Existential Medicine and Adjunct Fellow in Disruption. Behind him glowed a slide of a serene humanoid robot holding a stethoscope.

"Colleagues," he began solemnly, "we are here to confront an uncomfortable truth. AI is now better than many of us at diagnosing, reading scans, answering portal messages, writing insurance appeals, triaging GERD, detecting subtle ECG patterns, and possibly — " he paused for effect, " — expressing empathy."

A murmur rippled across the auditorium.

Somewhere in the back row, someone whispered, "Did a chatbot write this?"

Dr. Vector clicked to the next slide.

"Let us consider the vanguard. There are internists who now rehearse end-of-life conversations with chatbots. They practice inserting feeding tubes in simulated empathy before doing so in real life."

A hand shot up.

Dr. Maxwell Torque, an emergency physician whose badge read *Natural Intelligence Advocate*, stood without waiting to be recognized.

"I use AI all the time," he declared. "To *organize* my thoughts. Not to *think* them. I find it incorrect, invalid, and off point at least half the time. If someone needs a bot to tell a dying patient they have six months to live, perhaps they are in the wrong profession."

Applause erupted from the "NI Caucus," a loosely organized coalition of clinicians who preferred their cognition unassisted and their empathy unsimulated.

Dr. Vector adjusted his glasses.

"Some cardiologists and digital strategists believe AI's reasoning already outpaces physicians. They envision algorithms handling triage, interpretation, and counseling. Some have founded companies. Some advise them. Some do both."

From the second row, Dr. Prudence Quill, internist and part-time skeptic, leaned into the microphone.

"It's disappointing slop," she said evenly. "Grandiose claims. Financial conflicts. A narrative that human interaction is so complicated we need ChatGPT to rehearse it."

She looked around.

"No dystopian future required. We're already living in one."

Someone in Orthopedics coughed approvingly.

Dr. Crispin Heartwell, emergency physician and part-time philosopher, approached the podium for a counterpoint.

"We already have a model," he said. "Automated ECG readings. Good clinicians read the strip first. Then they look at the machine. If they agree, fine. If they disagree, reassess."

He gestured to the robot slide.

"AI excels at statistical consensus. We excel at nuance, smell, eye contact, and knowing when the patient says 'dizzy' but means 'the room is spinning and my left arm is weak.'"

A neurologist in the audience nodded vigorously.

"The art of medicine," Dr. Heartwell concluded, "is individuation. The science is statistical. Let's not confuse the two."

He paused.

"And if administration uses AI to give us 'cognitive breathing room' only to increase business targets, then the real diagnosis isn't AI — it's exploitation."

Thunderous applause. Even the robot on the screen seemed to blink.

Dr. Vector resumed.

"Consider the gastroenterologist who created a triage chatbot to filter reflux patients. He now sees fewer cases — but the complex ones. He predicts that when the algorithm outperforms him, he may need to 'find something different to do.'"

From the audience, Dr. Soren Vale, gastroenterologist and part-time nihilist, sighed.

"Wonderful. I've trained fifteen years so a bot can prescribe omeprazole."

A family physician shouted from the back:

"What we need is MORE DOCTORS. Not more bots. I need time — time to ask questions, time to notice subtle signs and symptoms. The patient has the answer. A chatbot doesn't."

The room hummed with agreement.

After a "mindful integration break" in which half the room lined up for coffee while loudly denouncing artificial intelligence and the other half quietly asked their phones to summarize the morning's arguments, the workshop segment followed: **Practicing Hard Conversations with Generative Empathy™**.

Participants were invited to pair off with tablets.

Dr. Helena Ward, internist, crossed her arms.

"If a doctor can't talk to a dying patient better than a bot," she said, "they have no business in patient care."

She refused the tablet.

"I didn't go into medicine to outsource compassion."

A psychiatry colleague leaned over and whispered, "I use it to draft termination letters so I don't sound angry. That's about it."

The psychiatrist next to her nodded.

"And patient handouts. It's fine for that."

A murmur of practical concession moved through the room.

Mid-symposium, the Wi-Fi flickered.

The robot slide froze, somewhere between a nod and a blink.

Dr. Bennett Slate, psychiatrist and part-time doom prophet, stood.

"What happens," he asked quietly, "when the internet isn't working?"

Silence.

The cardiology fellow clutched his phone reflexively.

Somewhere, a nurse practitioner whispered, "Does anyone remember how to auscultate without an app?"

The afternoon session turned darker.

Dr. Orion Fields, health systems researcher, addressed the crowd.

"AI can expand access. It can triage, reduce specialist bottlenecks, and remind us about screening guidelines."

He paused.

"But it can also recreate institutional bias. Pay less attention to women. Penalize spelling errors. Optimize billing instead of care."

A murmur of discomfort.

"AI deployed to optimize a broken system," he continued, "does not fix the system. It accelerates it."

A hospital administrator in the back scribbled "Efficiency Gains?" in her notebook.

During Q&A, a senior radiation oncologist took the microphone.

"I have zero concern that AI will overtake a good physician. There's already a shortage. The real problem is young doctors treating medicine like an 8-to-4 job. Shift work. Rotating faces. Patients don't know who their doctor is anymore."

He looked at the robot.

"If we give that system AI, it becomes more mechanical, not less."

A resident muttered, "We'd settle for manageable call schedules."

An ophthalmologist raised his hand.

"My patients consult Dr. Google before they see me. They still come. They still want a human to look them in the eye," pun intended, of course.

He smiled.

"And they still pay."

Laughter broke the tension.

An elderly primary care physician added:

"Even if AI has read all the literature, I'll still be sitting on a little rolling stool, talking to my patient. I'll still know their spouse's name, if I don't forget mine"

The image landed: the rolling stool as the last bastion of truth and humanity.

As the day wound down, Dr. Vector returned for closing remarks.

"So," he asked, "what are doctors really good for?"

From the back, Dr. Torque called out:

"Thinking."

Dr. Ward added:

"Feeling."

Dr. Heartwell:

"Integrating."

Dr. Vale:

"Questioning the premise."

The psychiatrist who used AI for termination letters shrugged.

"Editing."

Laughter again.

Finally, the neurologist who had spoken little all day stood.

"AI matches patterns," he said. "We extract meaning. AI predicts probabilities. We negotiate values. AI does not sit with fear."

He looked around the auditorium.

"The existential threat isn't that AI is better than us. It's that administrators will decide it's cheaper."

The room fell quiet.

Somewhere in the hallway, the Wi-Fi reconnected. Phones buzzed. An alert announced a new venture funding round for "Medical Superintelligence for Doctors."

Dr. Vector closed his laptop.

"Medicine is going to change," he said.

"Yes," Dr. Torque replied. "But we don't have to surrender our brains to prove we're modern."

As the physicians filed out, one resident paused beside the frozen robot slide and snapped a photo.

Caption: *Grand Rounds. Topic: Natural Intelligence.*

And somewhere, perhaps in Silicon Valley, an algorithm updated its model — learning that when physicians gather in a room and talk about being replaced, what they are really doing is reaffirming what cannot be downloaded:

A look in the eye.

A hand on the shoulder.

A question asked at just the right time.

No chatbot required.

* * *

Author's Note:

No chatbots were harmed in the writing of this satire.

The views expressed by the fictional physicians of St. Swithin's Medical Center are composites — an amalgam of real tensions currently animating medicine: awe, irritation, skepticism, pragmatism, entrepreneurial enthusiasm, and the lingering suspicion that if AI truly frees up our time, someone will promptly schedule another patient in it.

The intent here is not to caricature innovation nor canonize nostalgia, but to capture a moment in professional identity formation. Medicine has survived the stethoscope, the EKG machine, the CT scanner, the EHR, and Dr. Google. It will likely survive Dr. Chatbot as well.

Whether we emerge more human or merely more efficient remains a matter not of code, but of choice.

Section IV.

Systems, Policy, and the Future of Medicine

ESSAY 32.

Is AI Failing Healthcare, or Is Healthcare Failing AI?

THE EASY HEADLINE is that artificial intelligence is failing healthcare:

- A chatbot misses a triage cue.
- An ambient scribe inserts an error.
- A radiology algorithm performs admirably in a research study and disappoints in practice.
- A startup makes a grandiose claim, then a hospital embarrassingly shelves the product six months later.

The story almost writes itself: AI overpromised, underdelivered, and wandered into medicine before it was ready.

There is truth in that narrative. Some tools are bad. Some claims are absurd. Some medical AI products are built on narrow data sets, tested in artificial conditions, and marketed with a confidence that the evidence does not deserve. In medicine, hype is not harmless. A photo app with "bugs" is an inconvenience. A buggy clinical tool can distort care.

And yet, if we step back from the headlines, a more uncomfortable possibility emerges. Often, AI is not failing healthcare nearly as much as healthcare is failing AI. That does not mean the technology is innocent. It means the system into which it is being dropped is siloed, strapped, under-governed, and too often unprepared to absorb it safely. In other words, medical AI does not enter an innocent environment.

The Algorithm Is Rarely Alone

One of the most useful insights to come out of recent conversations about healthcare AI is that failure is rarely located in one place. It is rarely just the model. It is rarely just the hospital. It is rarely just the vendor. It is the interaction within a patchwork system.

A tool may perform well in development and fail in deployment. A hospital may want innovation but lack the data continuity, workflow discipline, or governance infrastructure to support it. Engineers may build something technically impressive without understanding the clinical moment in which it must actually function. Clinicians may distrust a tool not because they are anti-technology, but because they have seen too many systems arrive with fanfare and leave behind more work than they remove.

So, the question is not simply whether AI works. The better question is whether the surrounding system can carry it.

Workflow Is Not an Afterthought

One reason AI struggles in healthcare is overwhelmingly obvious: Many tools do not fit the workflow. They interrupt rather than support. They add clicks instead of removing them. They surface information without clarifying what action should follow. They arrive at the wrong moment, in the wrong format, to the wrong person.

This sounds mundane, but it is not. In clinical medicine, timing and fit are often the difference between usefulness and irrelevance. A model that detects a risk signal with impressive accuracy is not necessarily helpful if that signal appears after the physician has moved on, if no one owns the response, or if the interface requires an already overwhelmed clinician to open another tab, reconcile another summary, or verify another block of machine-generated text.

Healthcare has a long history of digitizing bad processes instead of redesigning them. AI risks becoming the newest layer on top of that old mistake. We cannot simply insert intelligent tools into unintelligent workflows and call it transformation. If a tool slows clinicians down, creates ambiguity, or increases cognitive burden, it will fail in practice, no matter how sound the model behind it may be.

Governance Cannot Begin After Deployment

Another recurring problem is governance. In too many organizations, governance is treated as something that happens after the tool is purchased, installed, and already influencing care. But in medicine, accountability is not optional.

- Who monitors performance over time?
- Who detects drift?
- Who reviews errors?
- Who decides when a tool is being over-relied upon?
- Who is responsible when the model output is wrong and the clinician is left holding the bag?

Hospitals know how to govern drugs, devices, credentials, infection control, and incident reporting. Yet AI often arrives in a gray zone — part IT purchase, part operations project, part clinical intervention, part vendor promise. That ambiguity is dangerous.

A low-risk documentation aid is not the same thing as a decision-support tool. A workflow assistant is not the same thing as a diagnostic model. A patient-facing chatbot is not the same thing as an imaging classifier. These systems do not carry the same risk and should not be governed as though they do.

Healthcare is not failing AI only by being slow or skeptical. It is also failing it by not building governance structures specific enough to match the kind of AI being deployed.

The Lab Is Not the Hospital

Then there is evaluation. Much of medical AI is still judged in settings that flatter it:

- Curated data sets.
- Exam-style questions.
- Retrospective analyses.
- Controlled environments with clean labels, stable inputs, and none of the mess that characterizes actual clinical care.

Real medicine is something else entirely. An AI tool must behave reliably in the noisy, time-pressured, causally tangled reality of care. This is why the real test of medical AI is not benchmark performance alone. A model can look superb on the Nürburgring and still struggle on a pothole-ridden road. Passing a test is not the same as surviving practice. Too often, we confuse research readiness with clinical readiness.

Data Quality Is Not Just a Technical Problem

There is another reason healthcare may be failing AI: the data itself. If patient identity is inconsistent, if documentation practices vary wildly, if coding is incomplete, if records remain split across institutions, then the AI layer built on top of that foundation will inherit those weaknesses. Garbage in, garbage out was true before machine learning (refer to Essay 14), and it remains true now. The difference is that AI can intensify the consequences.

Models trained in one geography may not generalize to another. Tools built from narrow data sets may behave unpredictably across different populations, resource settings, or disease patterns. Some systems are trained on data that are technically sufficient for publication but clinically insufficient for deployment.

Healthcare likes to imagine data as raw material waiting to be mined. In reality, healthcare data are a social artifact: disorganized, inconsistent, incomplete, shaped by billing rules, workflow shortcuts, human fatigue, local habits, and institutional priorities. That is not merely a machine learning challenge. It is a system challenge.

This Is Also a Collaboration Problem

One of the most revealing insights in discussions about healthcare AI is that different professions see different failure points.

Clinicians see work slowdowns and risks to patients. Operations leaders see fragmented processes and system unreadiness. Governance specialists see traceability and accountability gaps. UX researchers see products built without users. Data experts see continuity and representativeness problems. Patients see exclusion and mistrust. Builders see integration and adoption problems. Skeptics see hype outrunning evidence.

They are all partly right. No single profession sees the full picture. It is the old story of the blind men and the elephant: each grasps a piece and mistakes it for the whole.

That may be the true lesson: The failure of AI in healthcare is not only a technology problem or a healthcare problem. It is a collaboration problem. We keep trying to solve a socio-technical challenge from inside professional silos. The model is not enough. The hospital is not enough. The clinician is not enough. The vendor is not enough. Medical AI succeeds only when those worlds are designed to meet.

And Yet Some AI Really Is Failing Healthcare

To say healthcare is failing AI is not to absolve AI. Some tools are genuinely poor. Some are built by teams with little understanding of how healthcare works. Some are wrappers around opaque systems marketed with the confidence of a miracle drug and the evidence base of a slide deck. Some are tested in ways that amount to investor theater more than clinical science. Some are launched with the Silicon Valley assumption that one can ship early and fix later.

In medicine, "beta" is not a charming phase. It can be a patient. So the better formulation may be that AI is sometimes failing healthcare; healthcare is often failing AI; but most of all, we are failing to build the bridge between them.

What Would Success Look Like?

If AI is to succeed in healthcare, it must be treated less like a consumer technology and more like a medical intervention. That means:

- Designing around real clinical abrasion, not imagined user stories.
- Involving clinicians early, not after procurement.
- Separating low-risk workflow tools from high-risk clinical systems in governance.
- Stress-testing models on dirty, incomplete, real-world data.
- Measuring not just accuracy, but workflow fit, trust, edit burden, and actionability.
- Building accountability frameworks before deployment, not after harm.
- Monitoring performance over time, as we would with any intervention that can drift.
- Designing not only for hospitals and clinicians, but for patients and their uneven digital literacy.
- Insisting on transparency about training data, validation populations, and failure modes.

- Accepting that some AI belongs in healthcare now, while some does not.

And above all, it means abandoning the fantasy that the algorithm alone is the story.

A Stress Test for the System

Perhaps AI in healthcare should be understood not only as a tool, but as a stress test.

It exposes where workflows are brittle.

It exposes where ownership is unclear.

It exposes where documentation is incoherent.

It exposes where governance is performative.

It exposes where a hospital wants the prestige of innovation more than the discipline of implementation.

In that sense, AI does not merely enter the system. It reveals the system. That is why the question "Is AI failing healthcare, or is healthcare failing AI?" is so useful. It forces us to stop treating the model as a magical object — either savior or villain — and start examining the environment around it.

My own answer is that the latter is often closer to the truth. Not always. Not entirely. But often enough to justify action, to stop asking it to perform inside workflows that were never designed for it, under governance structures that remain underdeveloped, using data ecosystems that are fissured, in institutions that still confuse adoption with readiness.

The problem, then, is not just the technology. It is the system that keeps asking for transformation while resisting redesign. If AI is going to help medicine, healthcare will have to do something other than buying better models. It will have to become a better host.

Essay 33.

Can AI Fix a Broken Healthcare System?

Every few weeks, a new headline appears declaring that artificial intelligence will finally fix healthcare.

AI will reduce costs.
AI will eliminate diagnostic error.
AI will personalize treatment.
AI will relieve physician burnout.
AI will democratize access to care.

The promise is incredibly appealing. In a system widely acknowledged to be expensive, disjointed, and administratively bloated, the idea that a powerful new technology might rescue us is alluring. The underlying question is whether artificial intelligence is a true structural solution or merely a technologically sophisticated bandage applied to deeper wounds.

The Seduction of Technological Rescue

Artificial intelligence has genuine transformative potential. Some envision a near-future hospital visit that looks very different from today. A patient arrives, and the system instantly integrates their medical history, genomics, and population data to guide diagnosis and treatment. Redundant testing disappears. Personalized therapies replace trial-and-error prescribing. Clinical teams spend less time on paperwork and more time caring for patients.

Artificial intelligence could help bring parts of that vision into reality. But the phrase "could help" should be emphasized. Because even its most enthusiastic proponents acknowledge a critical limitation: Technology alone cannot repair a system whose underlying structure is flawed, and operations are dysfunctional.

The American healthcare system did not become dysfunctional because it lacked data processing power. It became dysfunctional because of structural incentives. Payment systems reward volume more than outcomes. Administrative complexity absorbs enormous resources, with some estimates suggesting there are now approximately 10 administrators for every 1 physician in the United States.[1] Insurance design often silos care. Prevention and long-term management are frequently undervalued.

Artificial intelligence cannot fix these structural problems by itself. While AI may revolutionize drug discovery, clinical trials, and personalized treatment planning, it cannot transform U.S. healthcare without fundamental reforms to infrastructure, payment systems, and clinical workflows. The most advanced algorithm cannot compensate for a system designed around misaligned incentives. Without reform, AI may simply accelerate the existing dysfunction.

The EHR Lesson

When electronic health records were widely adopted following the HITECH Act of 2009, the technology was supposed to improve efficiency, safety, and coordination. Instead, the early years of EHR implementation created an administrative burden that many physicians still struggle with today. Documentation requirements multiplied. Workflows were interrupted. Physicians spent hours navigating interfaces designed primarily for billing rather than patient care. The technology itself was not inherently flawed. But it was introduced into a system whose priorities were already distorted.

Artificial intelligence risks repeating that pattern. If deployed primarily to optimize billing, automate prior authorization battles, or accelerate claim denials, AI could deepen the administrative arms race between providers and payors rather than improving patient care. Indeed, early signs of this technological tug-of-war are already emerging: insurers using AI to scrutinize claims, physicians using AI tools to justify medical necessity, and both sides investing in algorithmic defenses. The result is not better care. It is faster bureaucracy.

Medicine has seen this movie before, and a remake is underway: *Suck It Up, Buttercup*.[2] The movie's website informs viewers: "Whether you're a clinician running on fumes, a patient who's been dismissed, or someone who simply believes healthcare should work for people, you're not alone."

Where AI Actually Helps

That does not mean AI is irrelevant to healthcare reform. Quite the opposite. As discussed in previous essays, artificial intelligence can make meaningful contributions in several domains where the system's complexity overwhelms human capacity. Here is a recap:

Administrative simplification.

Eligibility verification, claim submission, coding review, and error detection could be automated in ways that reduce clerical work for clinicians.

Clinical decision support.

AI-assisted tumor boards, diagnostic tools, and predictive models can help clinicians synthesize complex evidence more quickly.

Drug discovery and research acceleration.

Machine learning models can narrow the search space for new therapies and identify promising biological targets.

Personalized medicine.

AI can integrate genetic, clinical, and imaging data to guide individualized treatment strategies.

These are real advances. But notice something important: none of them addresses the fundamental economic architecture of healthcare. They make the existing system more efficient. They do not necessarily make it more rational.

Incentives Still Rule the System

The dominant payment model in the United States remains fee-for-service, which rewards volume of care rather than long-term health outcomes. In such a system, technologies that increase throughput often flourish more easily than those that prevent disease. For example, continuous monitoring, early detection, and preventive interventions may save lives and reduce long-term costs, yet reimbursement structures frequently fail to support these approaches.

Artificial intelligence cannot correct this imbalance on its own. If anything, it may create a greater divide. AI tools deployed in a volume-driven system may simply help deliver more billable services more efficiently. Technology follows incentives. It rarely rewrites them.

The Training Gap

There is also a cultural challenge. Medicine has always struggled with what researchers call the "know–do gap." On average, it can take more than a decade for evidence-based innovations to become standard practice. Artificial intelligence may widen that gap unless clinicians are properly trained to use it.

Integrating AI literacy into medical education, residency training, and continuing professional development will be essential. Physicians will need to understand how algorithms work, where they fail, and how to interpret machine-generated recommendations critically. Without that foundation, AI simply becomes another dense layer in clinical decision-making.

The Trust Problem

Perhaps the most fragile element of AI adoption in healthcare is trust (refer to Essay 29). Physicians want transparency about how algorithms generate recommendations. Patients want assurance that AI tools are safe, equitable, and subject to human oversight.

Public skepticism remains substantial. Surveys suggest that many patients feel uncomfortable with AI making diagnostic or treatment decisions.

Trust cannot be engineered purely through technical performance. It must be built through transparency, accountability, and meaningful human oversight.

A Tool, Not a Cure

Artificial intelligence may become one of the most powerful tools medicine has ever developed. It can expand diagnostic insight, accelerate discovery, and reduce administrative burden. Used wisely, it could help clinicians navigate the complexity of modern medicine more effectively. But expecting AI to "fix" healthcare misunderstands the nature of the problem.

The American healthcare system is not broken because it lacks computational power. It is broken because of incentives, fragmentation, regulatory complexity, and competing institutional priorities.

Artificial intelligence may help treat some of the symptoms. But unless the underlying structure changes, it will remain what many transformative technologies eventually become in healthcare: not a cure, but a sophisticated bandage useful mainly for the short-term, to buy time. They prevent deterioration. They allow healing to begin. But they are not the same as repair.

REFERENCES

1. Skibet C. 10 for every 1: when administrators outnumber the healers. SoMeDocs. July 20, 2025. https://doctorsonsocialmedia.com/10-for-every-1/.
2. Ellington K, Goldstein JA, McDermott N, McDermott R, Mulligan T, *et al.* *Suck It Up, Buttercup*. [Film]. American Academy of Emergency Medicine; 2026. https://siubfilm.com/.

Essay 34.

Autoland Is Not a Diagnosis: Rethinking the Aviation Metaphor for AI in Medicine

The pilot of a commercial aircraft, descending into near-zero visibility, hands control to an automated landing system ("autoland") designed precisely for that moment. The landing is flawless. The passengers are safe. The pilot announces it proudly. Technology performs exactly as intended.

A physician on board later reflects:

"It made me think about the healthcare journey I am on with AI. The safety and well-being of 140 people wasn't left to human intervention; the stakes were too high, and clearly, the machine has been proven to outperform humans. I wonder how long it will be before the trickiest diagnosis, the earliest detection, or the best recommendations are handled by the medical profession the same way my landing was?"

It is an elegant metaphor. It is also a dangerous one, at least when imported wholesale into medicine.

The Limits of the Aviation Analogy

In aviation, autoland serves a narrow, clearly defined purpose. The runway is fixed. The physics are stable. The environment is standardized. The system has been tested under rigorously controlled conditions. And crucially, it does not replace the pilot. It is used rarely, only under explicit rules, with oversight before, during, and after deployment. Fewer than 1% of landings rely on full autoland, not because the technology is inadequate, but because the system in which it operates is tightly bound and disciplined.

Medicine is none of those things.

The optimism embedded in the physician's reflection assumes that medicine's hardest moments resemble a fogbound runway — rare, well-defined, and ultimately solvable through sufficient data and algorithmic refinement. But the most difficult clinical problems are not low-visibility landings. They are ambiguous, evolving human situations in which even the destination may be contested.

A diagnosis is not a runway. A patient is not a system state. Clinical care is not governed by invariant physical laws.

The Complexity of Care

When aviation automation fails, investigations often trace the cause to identifiable categories: sensor malfunction, training error, software edge case, or interface breakdown. When medicine fails, the causes are rarely so discrete. They include social determinants, access barriers, trust, bias, timing, fear, financial constraint, and uncertainty itself. These are not variables to be filtered out. They are the substance of care.

The analogy also obscures a fundamental difference: who builds and governs the system. Aviation automation emerged within a tightly regulated industry shaped by decades of accident investigation, standardized aircraft design, and a global safety culture. By contrast, many medical AI systems are trained on incomplete data sets and developed within commercial ecosystems that reward speed and scale. Their incentives are not always aligned solely with safety. The sky in which they fly is not unbiased.

What Does "Outperform" Mean?

When an AI system is said to "outperform" a clinician, the claim requires scrutiny. Outperform on which population? Under what conditions? Using which definition of success?

A technically correct diagnosis delivered too late, or without the patient's trust, may still represent clinical failure. Medicine cannot be reduced to touchdown metrics.

Accountability further complicates the picture. When an aircraft lands itself, responsibility remains clear: The airline, manufacturer, regulators, and pilot operate within defined chains of oversight. In medicine, responsibility becomes diffuse as autonomy increases. If an algorithm misses an early cancer because its training data underrepresented a population, who answers to the patient? The clinician who relied on it? The institution that purchased it? The company that built it?

The algorithm cannot explain itself. It cannot apologize. It cannot assume liability. Yet its recommendations may feel authoritative, even when the reasoning is opaque.

Augmentation, Not Abdication

The vision of physicians proudly announcing that the "trickiest diagnosis" will now be handled by AI — like an autoland — rests on a false premise: that authority can be transferred without transferring understanding.

Patients do not seek pattern recognition alone. They seek interpretation, judgment, and partnership. They bring stories that do not fit neatly into training sets and fears that no model can quantify. They need someone to recognize when the data are technically correct but clinically incomplete.

There is no equivalent in medicine to "near-zero visibility at the field," a moment when the human should step aside because the machine sees better. There are moments when AI can assist in detecting patterns earlier, flagging risks, and managing complexity. Those contributions are real and worth embracing. But full autopilot in medicine would not represent augmentation. It would represent abdication.

A Better Aviation Lesson

If aviation offers a metaphor worth borrowing, it is not autoland. It is the pilot who understands automation deeply, who knows when to trust instruments and when to question them, who remains responsible even when the system is engaged.

Medicine does not need fewer humans at the controls. It needs clinicians who understand both the capabilities and the limitations of AI, who can interpret its outputs, challenge its assumptions, and integrate its guidance into the broader human context of care.

Safety in aviation has never depended on turning pilots into passengers. It has depended on understanding intricacy, designing for failure, and maintaining clear accountability. The same will be true in medicine. Planes do not heal people. Doctors do. And no degree of automation changes who must answer when something goes wrong.

Essay 35.

When the Machine Enters the Nursing Station: AI, Invisible Labor, and the Future of Doctor–Nurse Collaboration

For years, discussions about artificial intelligence in medicine have revolved around a dramatic question: *Will AI replace healthcare workers?* The more realistic question now surfacing is perhaps more consequential. What if AI does not replace clinicians at all, but instead reorganizes how their work is done?

A position statement from the American Academy of Nursing suggests that this process may already be underway.[1] The document offers one of the most detailed policy analyses to date of how AI could reshape nursing practice and clinical workflows across healthcare. What it reveals is less about technological triumph than about an evolving ecosystem of work, one that may subtly alter the relationships among clinicians, especially between nurses and physicians.

The Hidden Layer of AI in Clinical Work

Artificial intelligence has entered hospitals primarily through tools designed to make work easier:

- Ambient documentation systems.
- Predictive alerts.
- Triage algorithms.
- Workflow automation.
- Clinical decision support.

On paper, these tools promise efficiency. In practice, their effects can be more complicated. The nursing academy's statement notes that AI documentation tools, alert systems, and workflow automation may increase cognitive load, shift invisible labor onto clinicians, and introduce subtle forms of productivity surveillance if implemented without careful governance. These risks arise not from malice or poor engineering but from something more mundane: systems thinking.

Healthcare workflows are interconnected. When technology alters one task, the consequences ripple outward. A documentation tool that saves physicians time may require nurses to structure observations differently. An alert system that helps monitor patient deterioration may increase alarm fatigue on the floor. Automation that accelerates triage may redistribute decision-making responsibility in ways that no one anticipated.

None of these changes appears dramatic when examined individually. Together, they reshape the clinical environment.

The Rise of Invisible Labor

Nursing has always contained a large component of what sociologists call invisible labor. This includes tasks such as:

- Translating physician orders into bedside action.
- Coordinating care across multiple services.
- Monitoring subtle changes in patient condition.
- Mediating communication among clinicians, patients, and families.

These functions rarely appear in productivity metrics. Yet they are essential to safe care. AI systems may unintentionally shift more of this invisible labor downward in the hierarchy of healthcare work. Most healthcare AI does not remove work; it redistributes it.

A predictive monitoring system, for example, may generate earlier warnings about patient deterioration. That capability is clinically valuable. But responding to those warnings by validating them, documenting them, and escalating them often falls to nurses. Technology changes the signal. Humans still handle the response.

The Moral Tension of Machine Advice

Another emerging issue involves what happens when AI recommendations conflict with clinical judgment. Clinical decision-support tools increasingly offer risk predictions, triage recommendations, or treatment suggestions. Yet algorithms, like any model, operate on probabilistic reasoning derived from training data. Clinicians operate in a world of context and incomplete information.

The nursing academy's policy warns that when these two forms of reasoning diverge, clinicians may experience moral distress: the uncomfortable sense of knowing what one believes is the right course of action while facing pressure from institutional systems or technological outputs to do something different. This phenomenon is not theoretical. Anyone who has worked in a hospital has seen similar tensions with earlier technologies:

- Electronic health record prompts.
- Quality metrics.
- Clinical pathways.

AI simply intensifies the dynamic by adding an aura of algorithmic authority. When a screen suggests a course of action, disagreeing with it can feel like disobeying an authority figure.

AI as a System Architect

It is possible that focusing solely on clinician workload misses the larger transformation. Artificial intelligence does not merely assist individual tasks. It reshapes the flow of information, attention, and patients across the entire system. Consider triage algorithms used in emergency departments or telehealth systems. These tools influence:

- Which patients are flagged as high risk.
- Who receives early intervention.
- How resources are allocated.
- Which cases are escalated.

Over time, these decisions alter demand patterns across the healthcare system. Patient flow changes. Clinical priorities shift. Work is redistributed across departments and professions. The machine is not replacing clinicians. It is acting as a system architect.

The Economic Temptation

Hospitals operate on notoriously thin margins. In such an environment, any technology promising efficiency attracts attention from finance departments. If an AI system claims to reduce nursing workload by 20%, administrators inevitably ask the next question: What should we do with that 20%?

- Should staffing models change?
- Should positions be reduced?
- Should productivity expectations increase?

These are not cynical questions. They are economic ones. But they reveal a deeper tension in the deployment of healthcare AI. Efficiency gains can easily be translated into labor reductions rather than relational improvements in care. The nursing academy's policy implicitly warns against that possibility.

Protecting the Relational Core of Medicine

At its heart, nursing is a relational profession. The nurse–patient relationship involves observation, trust, and human connection — elements that cannot be fully captured in structured data. The policy emphasizes that AI must remain an adjunct to clinical judgment, not a replacement for it, and that human oversight should be embedded in all AI governance structures.

Equally important, the statement calls for mandatory workflow-impact assessments before AI deployment, ensuring that technology does not inadvertently undermine care processes or clinical relationships. This recommendation may prove more significant than it first appears. Healthcare organizations routinely conduct financial analyses before adopting new technologies. Far fewer evaluate how those technologies alter the lived experience of clinical work.

What This Means for Physician–Nurse Relationships

The physician–nurse partnership has always been central to hospital care. AI has the potential either to strengthen or strain that relationship. If implemented thoughtfully, technology could:

- Reduce documentation burden.
- Improve communication.

- Identify patient risks earlier.
- Free clinicians for more meaningful interactions.

But if implemented poorly, it could:

- Increase alarm fatigue.
- Redistribute administrative tasks.
- Create new hierarchies of algorithmic authority.
- Widen the gap between decision-making and bedside care.

In other words, AI may reshape not only how clinicians work, but how they work together.

The Governance Gap

Perhaps the most important observation emerging from current debates is this: Healthcare organizations carefully measure what AI does for efficiency. They rarely measure what AI does to clinicians.

- How does it change cognitive load?
- How does it redistribute responsibility?
- How does it alter professional relationships?

These questions rarely appear in implementation dashboards. Yet they may ultimately determine whether AI strengthens or weakens healthcare systems.

The Reorganization of Medicine

The American Academy of Nursing's policy statement does not reject artificial intelligence. On the contrary, it recognizes AI as a powerful force capable of improving care delivery. But it insists on something equally important: governance, transparency, and human oversight.

The debate about AI in healthcare has often been framed in dramatic terms: machines replacing doctors, robots running hospitals, algorithms diagnosing disease. The reality is subtler. AI is not replacing clinicians. It is reorganizing the work of medicine. And unless we measure those changes carefully, especially the invisible ones, the most profound transformation may occur not in the technology itself, but in the relationships that have long sustained the practice of care.

While much of what I have described in this essay will not strike readers as entirely new. Variations of these themes appear throughout this book and increasingly across the medical literature; the repetition itself carries meaning. When an idea begins to surface independently in multiple places, across professions and disciplines, it signals that something structural is shifting beneath the surface.

Physicians, nurses, informaticists, and policy leaders are beginning to describe the same phenomenon from different vantage points. AI is not simply adding a tool to clinical practice; it is rearranging the ecology of work inside medicine.

That convergence of concern is significant. It tells us that the issue is not technological hype or professional anxiety, but a genuine transformation in how care is organized, experienced, and governed. And if the reorganization is happening in different disciplines — through workflow changes, invisible labor, and subtle alterations in professional relationships — then noticing it, naming it, and discussing it repeatedly may be the first form of stewardship the profession can offer.

REFERENCE

1. American Academy of Nursing position statement on artificial intelligence in health care. American Academy of Nursing Press Release. March 16, 2026. https://aannet.org/news/722336/

Essay 36.

AI: Past, Present, and Future

Technological change in medicine is moving faster than any single observer can reliably forecast. New models appear almost weekly. Tools that seem revolutionary one month become obsolete the next. Entire categories of digital health products emerge, consolidate, and disappear within a few years. For that reason, I approach predictions about AI in medicine cautiously.

The End of the Pilot Era

For several years, health systems have experimented with artificial intelligence through pilot programs. A department deploys a predictive model. A startup installs a decision-support tool. A hospital tests an AI scribe or a revenue-cycle algorithm. Each effort produces promising results, but most remain isolated experiments.

Across the industry, hundreds of AI tools have been approved or cleared, yet relatively few have been integrated deeply into everyday clinical operations. The coming decade will likely mark the end of that experimental phase. Increasingly, health systems will be forced to move from curiosity to accountability. Leaders will ask difficult questions: What value did this system produce? Did it improve patient outcomes? Did it reduce administrative burden? Did it justify its cost?

The measure of success will no longer be whether artificial intelligence can perform a task. It will be whether organizations can use it responsibly, reliably, and widely.

Many industry observers already see this shift underway. Artificial intelligence is moving from isolated pilots to enterprise-level infrastructure, where its performance must be evaluated not only technically but operationally. This transition will separate the organizations that experiment with AI from those that actually benefit from it.

Technology Rarely Fails. Implementation Does.

One lesson has remained constant throughout my career. Technology itself rarely fails. Implementation strategy does. The temptation is to view artificial intelligence as a technological solution rather than an operational challenge. Leaders purchase software and expect transformation to follow automatically. But the real work begins after deployment.

Clinical workflows must change. Data governance must be strengthened. Staff must be trained. Accountability must be defined. Ethical oversight must be built into the process. Without those elements, even the most sophisticated algorithms become little more than digital curiosities.

The next decade in healthcare AI will not be won by organizations that deploy the most tools. It will belong to organizations that operationalize them intelligently, with more intelligence than the machines themselves claim to possess.

From Information to Understanding

For much of the digital health era, medicine focused on gathering data. Electronic health records digitized patient histories. Wearables tracked physiological signals. Imaging systems captured increasingly detailed visual information. Administrative databases recorded millions of transactions across the healthcare system. The result was not clarity. It was accumulation of data.

Clinicians today face unprecedented amounts of information, yet often struggle to locate the few facts that truly matter in a clinical decision. Artificial intelligence offers an opportunity to pivot from data accumulation to data interpretation.

In the coming decade, AI systems will increasingly operate across multiple forms of medical information simultaneously — text, voice, images, physiologic signals, and video. These systems will not merely store information but attempt to synthesize it, identify patterns, and surface insights that would otherwise remain buried within fragmented records.

In practical terms, this means clinicians may spend less time hunting for information and more time exercising judgment. If implemented carefully, such tools could reduce cognitive overload and restore attention to the human dimensions of care.

The Rise of Operational Intelligence

Artificial intelligence is often discussed in clinical terms: diagnosis, prediction, and treatment recommendations. Yet some of the earliest large-scale impacts may occur in areas that attract far less attention. Administrative tasks — documentation, scheduling, coding, billing, claims processing, care coordination — consume enormous resources across the healthcare system.

Many of these processes involve structured data, repetitive decisions, and pattern recognition, making them particularly well-suited to automation and machine learning. Improving these operational systems may not attract headlines, but the impact could be substantial.

When administrative processes become more efficient, clinicians regain time. When information flows more smoothly between systems, care coordination improves. When financial operations become more predictable, health systems can invest more consistently in patient care.

Artificial intelligence may not eliminate healthcare's complexity, but it can help make that complexity more manageable. In this sense, the true promise of AI may lie less in replacing physicians than in supporting the systems in which physicians work.

Trust Will Determine Adoption

Technology adoption in healthcare has always depended on trust. Physicians must trust that clinical tools are accurate and safe. Patients must trust that their information will be handled responsibly. Organizations must trust that systems will function reliably under real-world conditions. Artificial intelligence introduces new layers to that equation.

Models must be explainable. Data sources must be transparent. Governance structures must ensure accountability when errors occur. In the coming decade, one of the most important measures of AI success will be whether organizations can demonstrate that their systems are auditable, understandable, and trustworthy. Without that foundation, adoption will stall. With it, innovation can proceed more confidently.

The Physician's Role

Throughout this book, I have explored the unease many clinicians feel as artificial intelligence enters medical practice. Some view these technologies as threats. Others see them as tools. Most occupy a space somewhere in between.

Over the next decade, the physician's role will likely evolve in ways that resemble earlier technological transitions in medicine. When radiology adopted digital imaging, radiologists did not disappear. When electronic health records arrived, physicians did not become obsolete. Instead, clinicians adapted, sometimes reluctantly, to new forms of information and new methods of work. Artificial intelligence will follow a similar path.

Clinicians will increasingly interact with systems that summarize data, suggest possibilities, and highlight patterns. But the responsibility for judgment, including interpreting uncertainty, weighing context, and communicating with patients, will remain human. In fact, the more powerful the technology becomes, the more essential those human responsibilities may be.

Medicine has never been only about information. It has always been about meaning. That's what gave birth to the field of narrative medicine: the recognition that patients do not present as data sets but as stories, and that understanding those stories is itself a form of clinical knowledge.

A Cautious Optimism

Predicting the exact trajectory of artificial intelligence in healthcare would be foolish. The pace of change is simply too rapid. But some general conclusions seem reasonable.

Over the next decade, artificial intelligence will become embedded in the everyday infrastructure of healthcare organizations. Its greatest impact may emerge not through dramatic breakthroughs but through gradual improvements in workflow, coordination, and insight.

Health systems that approach AI thoughtfully, aligning clinical workflows, operational strategy, and governance around these technologies, will likely see meaningful gains in efficiency, quality, and sustainability. Those that treat AI as a collection of disconnected tools may struggle to realize its promise. The difference will not be the technology. It will be the discipline of implementation.

The future of medicine will not advance exactly as anyone imagines. Some innovations will disappoint. Others will exceed expectations. Many developments will surprise us entirely. Yet the broader direction seems clear. Medicine is entering an era in which intelligence — human and artificial — will increasingly operate together. The challenge for the next decade will not be deciding whether to use artificial intelligence. It will be deciding how to use it wisely. That task is distinctly human and belongs to us, not to machines.

Afterword

I HAVE LIVED THROUGH ENOUGH "next revolutions" in medicine to know that prediction is a fragile enterprise. The future rarely arrives as promised. It arrives altered by human behavior, by unintended consequences, and by the irreducible uncertainty of caring for patients whose stories never follow the script. Some forecasts prove spectacularly wrong, dismissed too quickly or embraced too soon.

Ignaz Semmelweis demonstrated in the 19th century that handwashing dramatically reduced maternal deaths. His colleagues rejected the evidence because it challenged prevailing assumptions about disease transmission. The pattern became known as the Semmelweis reflex: the instinctive rejection of new ideas that threaten established beliefs.[1]

Then there is Cassandra of Greek mythology, cursed to foresee catastrophe but never be believed. Her tragedy was not ignorance, but credibility.

Anyone writing about artificial intelligence in medicine risks becoming one or the other — dismissed as alarmist in the moment or overtaken by events that render today's certainties obsolete.

For that reason, this book has not attempted to predict AI's trajectory with precision. Instead, it explores something more immediate: what it feels like to practice medicine during a technological transition. These essays reflect on AI not as prophecy, but as lived experience — how it enters clinical spaces, reshapes professional roles, and alters the nature of daily work.

Across these essays, AI appears in many forms. It drafts clinical notes, summarizes research, analyzes imaging, suggests diagnoses, answers patient questions, and even generates language that approximates empathy. Each application promises efficiency, insight, and relief from administrative burden.

Yet the more resonant story is not technological. It is professional. Artificial intelligence compels medicine to revisit foundational questions: What counts as expertise? How does clinical judgment differ from statistical prediction? What responsibilities remain distinctively human in a profession increasingly assisted by intelligent systems?

In the coming decade, AI will almost certainly become more capable, more integrated, and more difficult to distinguish from human reasoning in certain domains. Algorithms will process medical data at scales no individual clinician can match. Systems will refine recommendations continuously, learning from vast data sets in ways that appear almost intuitive.

These advances are already reshaping how care is delivered. A large majority of physicians now use AI for documentation and communication tasks, signaling not a distant future but an ongoing transition. At the same time, the locus of care may shift. The patient's home, supported by wearable devices and remote monitoring, may increasingly function as clinic, observation unit, and even hospital, moving medicine away from episodic outpatient visits toward continuous, preventive care.

And yet, early experience offers a familiar lesson. Technology rarely fails in isolation; implementation does. Electronic health records promised efficiency and delivered documentation overload. Decision-support tools promised guidance and often produced alert fatigue.

This is the critical inflection point. Healthcare innovation — indeed, the future of medicine — may falter less from technical weakness than from misalignment: between tools and workflows, incentives and judgment, speed and reflection. Artificial intelligence will face the same test. It can strengthen the physician–patient relationship, or it can complicate it in ways that are subtle and cumulative.

Organizations that succeed in the age of AI will not simply deploy AI; they will operationalize it responsibly. They will align algorithms with clinical workflows, governance structures, and patient realities.

This is harder than it sounds. In business school, operations management is sometimes called the "organic chemistry" of management education, the discipline that reveals whether one truly understands how complex systems function. Many students resist it because it forces attention to process, sequencing, bottlenecks, and execution.

Healthcare is operations at its most intricate and least forgiving. AI will not simplify that complexity; it will expose it. Its success will depend less on computational brilliance than on disciplined integration, as shown in the accompanying figure.

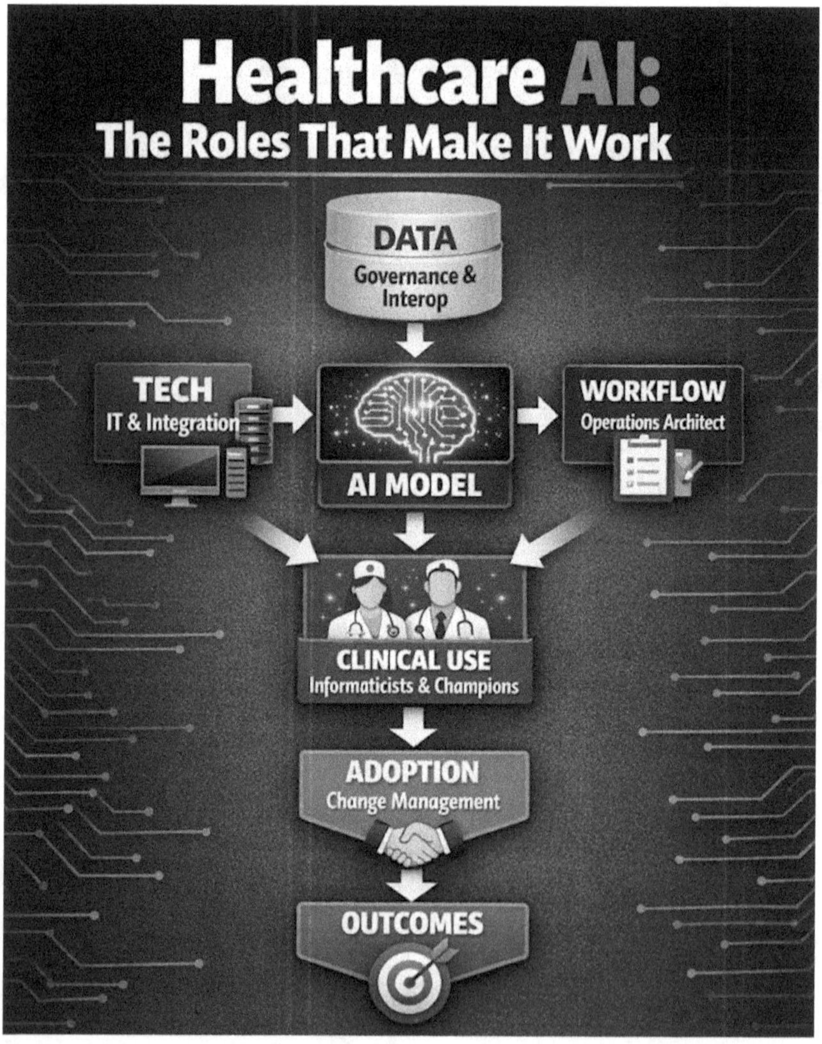

A recurring theme throughout this book is the evolution of physicians into editors of machine-generated knowledge. This shift is not merely technical. Editors do more than correct grammar. They safeguard accuracy, preserve meaning, and protect readers from careless error. In medicine, editorial responsibility translates into accountability for patient care.

AI can propose possibilities and identify patterns. It can even simulate empathic language. But it cannot assume responsibility for consequences. That obligation remains human.

This returns us to a central question proposed in the first essay in this book: whether the "A" in AI stands for Artificial or Augmented.

If AI is treated as a substitute for clinical judgment, it will eventually fail due to overconfidence, misuse, or misplaced trust. If it is used as augmentation, extending human insight while remaining subject to oversight, it may help address challenges that have long seemed intractable.

The next decade will reveal which path predominates. Some institutions will adopt AI hastily, propelled by financial pressure or technological enthusiasm. Others will resist reflexively, wary of disruption or erosion of professional authority. Both impulses are understandable. Both carry risk.

The more demanding course lies between them: deliberate adoption, critical scrutiny, and disciplined integration. It requires preserving the values that define medicine: curiosity, humility, compassion, and the willingness to question one's own assumptions in light of new evidence. It requires placing patient welfare above technological fascination. And it requires recognizing that no tool, however sophisticated, replaces the moral dimension of care.

Artificial intelligence will reshape documentation, research, diagnosis, and communication. It may even alter how medical knowledge is generated. What it should not alter is medicine's most basic commitment: to treat patients as individuals rather than data points, to listen for what is not said, and, above all, to serve the suffering rather than the system.

Machines may grow faster, more fluent, and more analytically powerful. But the future of medicine will still hinge on qualities they do not possess: judgment, empathy, and compassion.

Artificial intelligence will change how medicine is practiced. It cannot change why medicine is practiced.

That purpose remains uniquely ours.

REFERENCE

1. Lazarus A. *The Semmelweis Effect: When Medicine Knows Harm Exists — and Proceeds Anyway*. Self-published. 2026.

www.ingramcontent.com/pod-product-compliance
Lightning Source LLC
Chambersburg PA
CBHW071441230926
51846CB00001B/306
* 9 7 8 1 9 6 0 7 6 2 6 5 8 *